Food Fortification

Food Fortification
The evidence, ethics, and politics of adding nutrients to food

Mark Lawrence

Associate Professor and Director Food Policy Unit,
World Health Organization Collaborating Centre for
Obesity Prevention, Deakin University

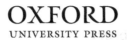

OXFORD
UNIVERSITY PRESS

OXFORD
UNIVERSITY PRESS

Great Clarendon Street, Oxford, OX2 6DP,
United Kingdom

Oxford University Press is a department of the University of Oxford.
It furthers the University's objective of excellence in research, scholarship,
and education by publishing worldwide. Oxford is a registered trade mark of
Oxford University Press in the UK and in certain other countries

© Oxford University Press 2013

The moral rights of the author have been asserted

First Edition published in 2013

Impression: 1

British Library Cataloguing in Publication Data
Data available

ISBN 978–0–19–969197–5

Printed and bound by
CPI Group (UK) Ltd, Croydon, CR0 4YY

Oxford University Press makes no representation, express or implied, that the
drug dosages in this book are correct. Readers must therefore always check
the product information and clinical procedures with the most up-to-date
published product information and data sheets provided by the manufacturers
and the most recent codes of conduct and safety regulations. The authors and
the publishers do not accept responsibility or legal liability for any errors in the
text or for the misuse or misapplication of material in this work. Except where
otherwise stated, drug dosages and recommendations are for the non-pregnant
adult who is not breast-feeding

Links to third party websites are provided by Oxford in good faith and
for information only. Oxford disclaims any responsibility for the materials
contained in any third party website referenced in this work.

Dedication

This book is dedicated to Anita, Sarah, and Robert:
you are constant sources of love, support, and inspiration.

Foreword

It is my pleasure to provide some introductory comments on this important piece of scholarship from Mark Lawrence. It seems almost too obvious to need to say that we should all do whatever we can to address malnutrition, and in particular undernutrition in children, that has such devastating long term consequences. The solution should most obviously be driven by a preventive public health approach to ensure children grow well and do not need to be 'treated'. Yet waiting until there is an acute problem does seem to be the norm before action begins. Starting from a public health or clinical treatment perspective makes a difference to the view as to how to address the problem; and acute needs usually take precedence over long-term solutions. But the on-going failure to build in prevention and to adopt a public health approach leads to the continuing need for an acute treatment model. So long term, ideally young women before they are pregnant and children in the first two critical years of life should have reliable access to enough good quality food, clean water, and basic health care needs. These are basic human rights. All agree, yet this does not seem to be enough to make it happen. Failure to address this is unacceptable.

In the context of this book, the question to address is what is the best way to ensure reliable access to enough good quality food to meet energy and nutrient needs. Over the last twenty years there has been a shift of emphasis away from social and community development driving a public health approach that seeks to ensure access to good quality food, to a more medicalized treatment approach which argues that it is not possible to ensure nutrient needs are met by diet alone. The preferred approach has been supplementation. At the same time, but with varying and uneven success and effort, fortification and plant breeding have also been worked on as ways to improve nutrient intakes. It is important to understand how this change in emphasis came about.

These important questions are at the heart of this very important book. For the first time, as far as I am aware, Mark Lawrence has set out in this book a rational framework for asking these questions and the scholarship in this book provides important answers.

This book is not a technical manual about how to do food fortification. This book is about more fundamental issues that need to be addressed before actually rushing into food fortification. Lawrence asks the big questions about food fortification: what are the public health benefits, risk, and ethical considerations of food fortification and alternative policy interventions; and how and why are food fortification policies made?

By using case studies within a conceptual framework the book reveals many important insights that, as far as I am aware, nobody else has previously uncovered about why food fortification is or is not used to address major public health nutrition problems. Key among these insights, for me, is that it is important to ask some basic questions as to what causes the problem fortification is seeking to address. If the problem is caused by a lack of a specific nutrient because of the degradation of the nutrient content of the soil in which a food is grown, or upon which animals graze, then it seems logical to seek ways to add that lost nutrient back into the food chain. If the aim of food fortification is to 'treat' a nutrient related medical problem, the symptoms rather than the cause, then there may be a different set of questions to ask as to whether fortification is the best way to address this problem. Mark Lawrence asks three important questions when assessing the appropriateness of food fortification policy: how to specify and measure public health risk; how to specify and measure ethical considerations; and how to compare scientific uncertainties and ethical considerations across the possible policy solutions against background plausible policy options. Thus, for each problem the key issues to consider are: what are the different policy options to address the problem; what are the public health benefits and risks for each option; and what are the ethical considerations for each policy option. In Section 2 of the book, Mark uses this framework in three case studies: universal salt iodization; mandatory flour fortification with folic acid; and mandatory milk fortification with vitamin D. For each case study in addition to using the above framework he also explores the actors, activities, and agendas that have been engaged in the area of work.

In the third and last section of the book, Mark Lawrence draws conclusions and provides some insights as to the way forward. One size does not fit all—the responses to key public health nutrition challenges need to be appropriate to the local circumstances that cause the problem. This requires scholarship at the local level to understand the problem and think about relevant and appropriate local solutions, particularly if the aim is to address local inequalities. Carrying on doing the same things in the same way as we are currently doing does not make a lot of sense. If the learning from this book is applied more widely we just may start to do things more effectively, or at the very least going about developing programmes based on some a priori logical framework for better decision making.

Barrie Margetts
Professor of Public Health Nutrition
Faculty of Medicine, University of Southampton
President, World Public Health Nutrition Association

Preface

In my academic role as a public health nutritionist, I am regularly confronted with the challenge that is food fortification and its advantages and disadvantages for public health. Students and the general public have long been advised by nutritionists that a healthy diet is one that conforms to the principles of balance, variety, and moderation. Yet, in contemporary times how relevant and accurate are these principles when one serve of a cereal product may be fortified to provide a novel variety of nutrients and in greater amounts than exists in a combination of foods from all other food groups? Does it matter if that cereal product is also 40% by weight added sugar?

As a member of the public and a parent, the challenges I face may be different but they persist. Governments around the world are regulating to varying degrees for the addition of iodine, folic acid, and vitamin D, among other nutrients, to staple foods in their country's food supply. It is increasingly likely that people in many countries now are consuming a diet that regularly contains at least one fortified food. These government activities are intended to provide public health benefits though they will provide little health benefit for my young children or myself and may confer some risk. Balancing the evidence for benefits and risks, struggling with ethical dilemmas, and negotiating the politics associated with the competing views of actors, are constant themes in food fortification. It is for this reason that this book is entitled *Food Fortification: The* Evidence, Ethics *and* Politics *of Adding Nutrients to Food*.

The idea for this book arose from my experiences with the evidence, ethics, and politics of food fortification from several perspectives. When I was the Acting Nutrition Director at the then Australia New Zealand Food Authority (now Food Standards Australia New Zealand), the Authority was immersed in two especially vexed food fortification debates—whether folic acid should be added to staple foods to help prevent neural tube defects (see Chapter 6), and whether food regulations should be relaxed to give food manufacturers more control over fortifying and marketing their products. As the Leader of the Australian delegation at a Codex (in effect the international food regulator) nutrition committee meeting I witnessed similar vexed food fortification debates at the global level and observed the power of certain food manufacturers in influencing these debates. In contrast, when working as a nutritionist in Pacific Island countries and Vietnam I have had the opportunity to be involved in projects in which food fortification has been a valuable policy option for tackling food security concerns.

The purpose of this book is to present the findings of original research into food fortification. The research aim was to provide insights into the public health benefits, risks, and ethical considerations of food fortification as well as understandings of its policy-making processes. It is intended that the achievement of this research aim will help students, practitioners, and policy-makers identify how food fortification policy processes and subsequent policy outcomes might be improved to further protect and promote public health.

A number of food fortification books are available. Typically the purpose of such books is to describe food fortification interventions and the various technical details such as the regulatory conditions under which fortification might occur. Other books (such as Allen L, de Benoist B, Dary O, Hurrell R (eds). *Guidelines on food fortification with micronutrients*. Geneva: World Health Organization and Food and Agricultural Organization; 2006. Available from: http://www.who.int/nutrition/publications/guide_food_fortification_micronutrients.pdf), provide practical guidance for designing and implementing food fortification programmes. These perspectives are important. However, they are not sufficient to gain an understanding of the interactions between evidence, ethics and politics that help elucidate the benefits, risks and ethical considerations associated with food fortification and how and why such policies are made.

The research presented in this book is cutting edge in that it helps fill this current gap in our understanding of food fortification. The research is up to date and peer-reviewed. To my knowledge it is the first food fortification investigation to strategically combine an evidence and ethics assessment with a critical analysis of food fortification case studies. The book introduces a novel conceptual framework that was used to systematically and robustly organize the research. It then presents the findings from combined assessment and critical analysis approaches that were used to investigate three topical food fortification case studies. Insights from the research are then identified and discussed.

The intended readership of the book is upper undergraduate- and postgraduate-level students enrolled in food and nutrition, public health, health promotion, dietetics, public policy, and medical courses, as well as practitioners in these disciplines, researchers and policy-makers.

Food fortification is a vast and diverse public health topic. This book does not attempt to provide a comprehensive assessment and analysis of all aspects of food fortification. Necessarily decisions had to be made about setting boundaries for the book's scope. Food fortification is predominantly of two types—mandatory food fortification and voluntary food fortification. This book's focus is on mandatory food fortification. This is because it is the food fortification type that is managed by government as a technology for the explicit purpose of promoting and protecting public health. This focus is not intended to diminish the public health implications of voluntarily fortified foods in the contemporary food supply.

Governments may propose voluntary food fortification as a policy option to tackle certain nutrition problems and this book does consider voluntary food fortification from this perspective. However, voluntary food fortification operates primarily to serve commercial objectives. Although governments regulate for voluntary food fortification, it is at the discretion of food manufacturers when, and to a large extent in what form, voluntary food fortification is implemented. Commonly it is high sugar- and salt-containing and low nutrient food and drink products such as refined cereals and juice drinks that are fortified on a voluntary basis.

The proliferation of voluntary fortified foods in the modern food supply introduces a different public health agenda to that for mandatory food fortification. Perversely, it is the addition of nutrients to these less healthy food products that then is exploited to trigger marketing claims suggesting that they have health promoting benefits despite their contribution to prevalent dietary imbalances threatening public health nutrition. An investigation of voluntary food fortification requires a separate research orientation to that presented in this book. Rather than investigating how food fortification might be used proactively to *promote* public health, research into voluntary food fortification might better be oriented towards investigating how to *protect* public health in response to commercial agendas for such fortification.

An activity that is frequently identified in the analysis of the case studies in this book is 'framing'. In this book framing refers to the process of giving meaning and legitimation to a policy problem and a proffered policy solution. Framing does not just relate to the activities of the actors involved in the case studies. As the author of this book my views are irrevocably present in how the research investigation for each case study was framed. Although my views could not be removed from the research processes, their potential influence could be managed. In addition to declaring the presence of my views in the research, two actions were undertaken to promote a balanced and objective approach to the case study investigations. First, the conceptual framework was applied to explicitly outline the logic that informed how the investigation was structured and the specific case studies were selected so as to each represent one of three plausible rationales for food fortification.

The second action was that when assessing and analysing the case studies at the heart of the research I attempted to represent all major views on a topic. It is widely accepted that universal salt iodization (USI) (Chapter 5) represents a well-substantiated case for mandatory food fortification and that is the predominant view presented for that case study. Alternatively, there is a diversity of views towards using food fortification as a policy intervention to address the policy problems of micronutrient malnutrition in its broad sense (addressed within the USI case study), neural tube defects (Chapter 6), and vitamin D deficiency (Chapter 7). In promoting balance in the investigation I present the range of views associated with these case studies. However, I do not resile from identifying scientific uncertainties and ethical dilemmas associated with the use of mandatory food fortification in each case study. Critically, I also draw particular attention to the existence of one or more 'complicating factors' associated with each of these more contested case studies. These complicating factors indicate that despite each of these food fortification case studies being associated with scientific uncertainties and ethical dilemmas, there is a reason for considering food fortification as a policy option. It is the existence of the complex mixture of scientific uncertainties, ethical dilemmas, and complicating factors that make each topic a particularly rich case study of food fortification.

The book has been written deliberately to challenge certain conventional views about food fortification that might be held by some readers. It seeks to encourage new ways of thinking about the role of this technology in promoting and protecting public health. It will have gone a long way to achieving its research aim if it succeeds in provoking readers to critically analyse what is happening with food fortification in countries around the world, how and why it is happening and what its public health benefits, risks and ethical considerations are.

Mark Lawrence

Table of contents

Acknowledgements

This book is the culmination of observations, experience, knowledge, and ideas generated over many years and involving numerous people. It has been enriched through the generous support, encouragement, and expert advice of many colleagues and friends including: Martin Caraher, John Coveney, Sharon Friel, Roger Hughes, Tim Lang, Anita Lawrence, Amanda Lee, Barrie Margetts, Kerin O'Dea, Christina Pollard, Mike Rayner, Rosemary Stanton, Boyd Swinburn, Mark Wahlqvist, Tony Worsley, Heather Yeatman, and my friend and mentor, Barbara Smith.

The quality of the book was strengthened significantly by the professional reviewing undertaken by Ian Darnton-Hill and Janine Lewis, both of whom are international experts in food fortification policy and practice.

I was fortunate to have excellent editorial support provided by Rebecca Reynolds and Karishma Kripalani who helped progress the book.

A particular note of appreciation to my colleagues in the Population Health Strategic Research Centre and the School of Exercise and Nutrition Sciences at Deakin University as well as the many students with whom I have had the opportunity to teach, discuss, and debate public health nutrition and food policy.

Finally, thank you to Nic Wilson, Caroline Smith, and Elizabeth Chadwick at Oxford University Press for their patience, advice, support, and more patience, throughout the book's preparation and production.

Note that the text excerpts below are kindly reproduced with permission as outlined:

> A problem has to be defined, structured, located within certain boundaries and be given a name. How this process happens proves crucial for the way in which a policy is addressed to a given problem. The words and concepts we employ to describe, analyse or categorize a problem will frame and mould the reality to which we seek to apply a policy or 'solution'. The fact that we may share the same data, or at least believe that we share the same data, does not mean that we shall see the same thing. Values, beliefs, ideologies, interests and bias all shape perceptions of reality.
>
> (Parsons, W. *Public policy: an introduction to the theory and practice of policy analysis.* Cheltenham: Edward Elgar Publishing Ltd, 1995.)

> ... public policy and the problems with which it is concerned do not exist in neat, tidy, academic boxes... the aim of the policy approach is not to pull these issues apart, so much as to recognize how problems come to be addressed and structured by the way

in which knowledge is organized and deployed... consequently and inevitably the study of policy-making and policy analysis is essentially multiframed.

> (Parsons, W. *Public policy: an introduction to the theory and practice of policy analysis*, Cheltenham: Edward Elgar Publishing Ltd, 1995.)

Are certain actors striking a correct balance in representing public health and commercial interests?: The job of government is to create the conditions that make it commercially viable for food companies to take up the challenge of VM (Vitamin and Mineral) deficiency. For example, governments can:

- Help build public demand for fortified foods through health and education services, and the print and broadcast media.
- Assist with start-up finance, technical training, product development, consumer testing, and marketing costs.
- Endorse approved food products, with official government seals or stamps for use in commercial advertising.
- Allow distribution of certain fortified foods via schools, hospitals, clinics.
- Specify fortified foods when placing food orders for schools, the armed forces, health service personnel, or for disaster relief and refugee feeding programmes.

These are the kind of public-private partnership deals can make it viable for food companies to invest in developing and marketing fortified products that will be available to the poor.

> UNICEF and the Micronutrient Initiative. *Vitamin and mineral deficiency: a challenge to the world's food companies*. Micronutrient Initiative, Ottawa; 2004. Available from: http://www.micronutrient. org/CMFiles/PubLib/Report-70-VMD-A-chanllenge-to-the-Worlds-Food-Companies1NMP-3242008-7366.pdf (accessed 24 January 2012).

A RIS is mandatory for all decisions made by the Australian Government and its agencies that are likely to have a regulatory impact on business or the not-for-profit sector, unless that impact is of a minor or machinery nature and does not substantially alter existing arrangements. This includes amendments to existing regulation and the rolling over of sunsetting regulation.

> Department of Finance and Deregulation. *Best Practice Regulation Handbook*. Australian Government: Canberra, 2010. Available from: http://www.finance.gov.au/obpr/proposal/handbook/docs/ Best-Practice-Regulation-Handbook.pdf.

List of abbreviations

ACF	advocacy coalition framework	IOM	Institute of Medicine
AI	adequate intake	LMIC	low- and middle-income countries
BINGO	business interest non-government organization	MDGs	millennium development goals
CCNFSDU	Codex Committee on Nutrition and Foods for Special Dietary Uses	MFFFA	mandatory flour fortification with folic acid
CDC	Centers for Disease Control and Prevention	MI	Micronutrient Initiative
Codex	Codex Alimentarius Commission	MMFVD	mandatory milk fortification with vitamin D
EBM	evidence-based medicine	NGO	non-government organization
eLENA	electronic library of evidence for nutrition actions	NHD	Health and Development (WHO Department of)
eWG	electronic working group	NTD	neural tube defect
FAO	Food and Agriculture Organization	NUGAG	Nutrition Guidance Expert Advisory Group
FDA	Food and Drug Administration (US)	OBPR	Australian Department of Finance and Deregulation's Office of Best Practice Regulation
FFI	Flour Fortification Initiative	PINGO	public interest non-government organization
FSA	Food Standards Agency (UK)		
FSANZ	Food Standards Australia New Zealand	PPP	public–private partnership
GAIN	Global Alliance for Improved Nutrition	RCT	randomized controlled trial
GRADE	grading of recommendations, assessment, development, and evaluation	RDA	Recommended Dietary Allowance
		RIS	regulatory impact statement
HICs	high-income countries	SAC	school-age children
ICCIDD	International Council for the Control of Iodine Deficiency Disorders	SPS	agreement on sanitary and phytosanitary measures
IDD	iodine deficiency disorders	SUN	Scaling Up Nutrition
IDRC	International Development Research Centre	TBT	agreement on technical barriers to trade
		UIC	urinary iodine concentration
IFPRI	International Food Policy Research Institute	UL	tolerable upper intake level
		UN	United Nations
IMMPaCt	CDC's international micronutrient malnutrition prevention and control program	UNICEF	United Nations Children's Fund
		USAID	United States Agency for International Development

USI	universal salt iodization	WFP	World Food Programme
UVB	ultraviolet B	WHA	World Health Assembly
VDR	vitamin D receptor	WHO	World Health Organization
VMNIS	Vitamin and Mineral Nutrition Information System	WTO	World Trade Organization

Chapter 1

Introduction

The right to health means that governments must generate conditions in which everyone can be as healthy as possible. Such conditions range from ensuring availability of health services, healthy and safe working conditions, adequate housing and nutritious food (1, p. 1).

Food, nutrients, and health

Food is essential to life. It provides the nutrients necessary for growth, development, and health maintenance. Modern humans' nutrient requirements are an outcome of millions of years of evolution, as human physiology has adapted to available food supplies (2). Although it is not possible to be sure whether the amount and composition of available food supplies has been optimal for health as the environment changed over the centuries, it evidently has been adequate for human survival (at least until reproductive age). The relatively recent global epidemic of diet-related non-communicable diseases, such as cardiovascular disease, cancer, and type 2 diabetes, has been attributed in part to contemporary nutrient intake patterns that depart from those that have existed for much of human evolution along with social and environmental patterns, such as changes in physical activity. Specifically, it seems likely that the rate of change in nutrient intakes over the past several hundred years has occurred more rapidly than the genes that shape our physiology have been able to evolve and adapt (3).

Throughout history the inter-relationship between human physiology and available food supplies has taken place within an ecological setting that has mediated the availability and nutrient composition of individual foods. Then, as food science and technology skills developed, scientists gained the capacity to manipulate the compositional characteristics of certain foods. Almost 100 years ago food scientists, often in collaboration with nutritionists who had access to a rapidly growing nutrition knowledge base, began adding nutrients to certain foods as a technological intervention to support public health policy objectives or pursue commercial opportunities. The addition of essential nutrients to certain foods became known as food fortification.

What is food fortification?

Food fortification is defined by the Codex Alimentarius Commission (Codex), which is in effect the international food regulator (see Chapter 3), as '... the addition of one or more essential nutrients to a food whether or not it is normally contained in the food for the purpose of preventing or correcting a demonstrated deficiency of one or more nutrients' (5, p. 2). The Codex general principles for the addition of essential nutrients to foods were in the early stages of the Codex review process (4) at the time of writing, and so their 1991 version is used as the reference for food fortification principles in this book. These 1991 Codex principles state that the following conditions should be fulfilled for any fortification programme (5, p. 3):

> There should be a demonstrated need for increasing the intake of an essential nutrient in one or more population groups. This may be in the form of actual clinical or subclinical evidence of deficiency, estimates indicating low levels of intake of nutrients or possible deficiencies likely to develop because of changes taking place in food habits.

Food fortification is one of four purposes for adding nutrients to foods recognized by Codex, the other three purposes being (5, pp. 1, 2):

Restoration: 'The addition to a food of essential nutrient(s) which are lost during the course of good manufacturing practice, or during normal storage and handling procedures, in amounts which will result in the presence in the food of the levels of the nutrient(s) present in the edible portion of the food before processing, storage or handling'. For example, adding thiamin to flour to a level comparable to that originally present in the wheat grain before it was milled.

Achieving nutritional equivalence of substitute foods: where nutritional equivalence is defined as: 'Being of similar nutritive value in terms of quantity and quality of protein and in terms of kinds, quantity, and bioavailability of essential nutrients'. Substitute food is defined as: 'A food which is designed to resemble a common food in appearance, texture, flavour, and odour, and is intended to be used as a complete or partial replacement for the food it resembles'. For example, adding vitamin A to margarine in an amount equivalent to that present in butter, for which it is a food substitute.

Ensuring the appropriate nutrient composition of a special purpose food: where special purpose foods are defined as: 'Foods that have been designed to perform a specific function, such as to replace a meal, which necessitates a content of essential nutrients which cannot be achieved except by addition of one or more of these nutrients'.

This book focuses on food fortification, in particular mandatory fortification and to a lesser extent, voluntary food fortification. It briefly refers to the more specialized areas of biofortification of staple foods (the breeding and genetic modification of plants to improve nutrient content and/or absorption) and household fortification (adding nutrients in the form of tablets, powders, and spreads to foods at the household level). Mandatory and voluntary food fortification are broadly distinguishable in relation to who controls the decision to fortify a food. In the case of mandatory food fortification, governments set food law that obliges food manufacturers to fortify particular foods or categories of foods with specified nutrients, and often at specified levels. Generally, governments mandate food fortification in response to evidence that a public health problem has a high prevalence and/or high severity. In comparison, voluntary food fortification involves governments setting food law that specifies permissions within which food manufacturers can then choose whether or not to fortify particular foods. This latter policy approach may be recommended by governments as a more flexible alternative to mandatory food fortification when responding to a particular public health problem. However, typically food manufacturers take advantage of these permissions to pursue marketing opportunities, either by creating a new food product or to differentiate an existing food product from that of a competitor's.

The first mention of food fortification occurred in 400 BCE, when the Persian physician Melampus (medical advisor to Jason and the Argonauts) suggested that adding iron filings to wine would increase the 'potency' of soldiers (6). In more contemporary times, food fortification has been intertwined with the modern history of nutrition. It was during the so-called golden era of nutrition in the first half of the 20th century, characterized by the 'discovery', isolation, and elucidation of many nutrients, that the impetus for the evidence-informed addition of nutrients to certain foods was created. As food and nutrition science evolved, the growing technological capacity and evidence base fuelled the need for more investment into food fortification policy. Hence fortification progressively expanded to cover more nutrients, foods, public health problems, and marketing opportunities.

The first time food fortification was used as an evidence-informed public health intervention occurred in the early 1920s in Switzerland when table salt iodization to help prevent endemic goitre was introduced (7). The US closely followed (8). During this era, other nutrition-related conditions, including anaemia, beri beri, pellagra, and rickets, were also prevalent among many populations. Burgeoning knowledge regarding nutrient–health relationships and food composition, as well as surveillance to collect dietary intake data, provided insights into preventing these afflictions. In addition, technological developments in food science were opening up possibilities of enabling foods to be fortified with nutrients to help tackle these public health problems. Over the following 50 years, a number of food fortification public health programmes, mostly in industrialized nations, were implemented. The more prominent nutrient–food vehicle combinations during this period were: vitamin D-fortified milk, vitamin A-fortified margarine, and B-group vitamin- and iron-fortified flour.

Increasingly from the 1970s, food fortification programmes were introduced into low- and middle-income countries (LMICs) as a policy intervention to tackle micronutrient malnutrition. The magnitude of the problem of micronutrient deficiencies is substantial, and infants, children, and pregnant and lactating women are especially vulnerable. Globally, it is estimated that there are approximately two billion people whose diet lacks sufficient amounts of vitamins and minerals essential for health (9). More than a third of child deaths and more than 10% of total global disease burden is attributed to maternal and child undernutrition overall (10). Over the past 20 years in particular, there has been a concerted effort from United Nation (UN) agencies to highlight and address micronutrient malnutrition, and food fortification has received particular attention as a priority policy option (11, 12). Food fortification is a strategic initiative aligned with six of the eight Millennium Development Goals (MDGs). These goals were set at the UN millennium summit to guide international development work to help bridge the gap between rights and reality for the world's poor by the year 2015. In the context of progress towards the achievement of the MDGs, the UN Standing Committee on Nutrition has instigated its 'Scaling Up Nutrition' agenda to increase investment in food fortification (13).

Food is not just a public health resource, it is also big business. Global food retail sales are estimated to represent US$ four trillion annually (14). Fortified food products represent a significant component of this figure. A number of food manufacturers, located mainly in industrialized countries, are taking advantage of voluntary food fortification permissions to develop niche products and/or to differentiate their products according to the target market. Consequently, the modern food supply has a proliferation of voluntarily-fortified food products, notably in the categories of breakfast cereals, beverages, and dairy products. Powerful marketing opportunities arise when these voluntarily-fortified food products can be promoted with nutrition and health claims based on their nutrient content levels and novel nutrient composition. In addition, the suppliers of the fortificants that are essential ingredients for fortified foods are active participants in the food marketplace. For example, at its curiously titled website URL http://www.pourontheprofits.com (15), the prominent nutritional ingredient supplier, DSM, explicitly frames food fortification as a business opportunity.

The presence of fortified foods in the modern food supply

Fortified foods are ubiquitous in the modern food supplies of LMICs and high-income countries. The US Centers for Disease Control and Prevention reports that globally between 2004 and 2007, the percentage of roller mill-processed wheat flour that was fortified increased from 18% to 27% (see Figure 1.1). This is especially significant because wheat flour is the most consumed cereal flour in the world (16). This trend is gaining momentum and by the end of 2011 it was estimated that across the world 30% of the flour processed in large roller mills was fortified (17).

The extent of exposure to novel nutrient profiles varies among countries around the world. Across Europe, fortified foods are reported to not significantly contribute to nutrient intake levels (18). By contrast, some argue that if it were not for fortified foods and nutrient supplements, significant proportions of the

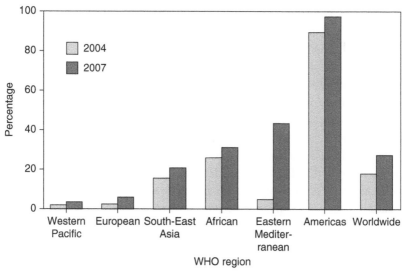

Fig. 1.1 Percentage of wheat flour processed in roller mills that was fortified: worldwide and by World Health Organization (WHO) region, 2004 and 2007.

Reproduced from G Maberly et al. Trends in wheat-flour fortification with folic acid and iron – worldwide, 2004 and 2007. *Morbidity and Mortality Weekly Report* (MMWR), 57(1): 8–10, Centers for Disease Control and Prevention (CDC), Copyright © 2008.

US population would struggle to achieve the US dietary reference intake for a number of micronutrients (19).

The growing proliferation of mandatorily- and voluntarily-fortified food products in the marketplace shows little sign of abating. At the time of writing, many technical, governance, and political developments are underway that are predicted to provide a strong platform to drive expanded food fortification policy and practice activities into the future. From a public health perspective, the World Health Organization (WHO) is building an evidence base to inform food fortification policy and practice decisions, as well as providing a range of resources to support food fortification programmes. These WHO activities are taking place at the same time as Codex is reviewing its general principles for the addition of essential nutrients to foods. Moreover, various partnerships and alliances are being formed to strengthen capacity to implement food fortification programmes, and national and regional level collaboration is facilitating the roll-out of such programmes (see Chapter 3).

It is not just mandatory food fortification programmes that will be driving an anticipated increased presence of fortified foods in the marketplace into the future. It is likely that the commercially-oriented motivation for and investment in voluntary food fortification also will continue to grow. Survey data published in the food marketing literature consistently report people's positive attitudes towards fortified foods, highlighting the commercial attractiveness of fortification. For example, the findings of one 2011 survey indicate that approximately 80% of the US adult population believe that fortification (and 'foods with added benefits') plays at least some role in their food purchasing behaviour, i.e. certain foods and beverages are purchased specifically because of a perceived added benefit of fortification (20). Moreover, according to the results of a 2010 survey of US adult primary grocery shoppers, fortification is a stronger influence on the perception of what is a healthy food than the removal of sugar, saturated fat, and sodium (21).

The extent of novel nutrient exposure in populations is increased when the availability of fortified foods is considered alongside the significant purchase and consumption of nutrient supplements among citizens in many countries. It is estimated that the value of the global market for vitamin supplements alone, i.e. not including mineral supplements, will reach US$ 3.3 billion by the year 2015 (22).

The contested nature of food fortification

The substantial presence of mandatorily- and voluntarily-fortified food products in the modern food supply represents a significant departure from the typical nutrient profiles that humans have been exposed to for most of recorded history. The net result is that the majority of the world's population is being exposed to unprecedented amounts and unusual combinations of nutrients. The health implications of these novel nutrient exposures are uncertain. As Jacobs and colleagues comment: 'The biologic systems involved in nutrition and disease are complex and not completely understood. We do know, however, that the human body did not evolve in the presence of a fortified food supply' (23).

As a technological intervention, food fortification is a particularly vexed and contested public health policy topic. Its ability to raise nutrient intakes across populations relatively extensively, rapidly, and cheaply, in combination with the way that many fortified food products are marketed, is considered as either a strength or a concern among actors in government, public health, and the private sector. In many areas food fortification has demonstrated impressive successes. However, there are also extraordinary claims made about food fortification and high expectations about its ability to solve dietary deficiencies and various other public health nutrition problems.

Proponents of food fortification point to its track record of having helped achieve many successful public health outcomes as well as its specific advantages as a public health intervention. Such advantages include its ability to passively increase the intake of a certain nutrient, 'or combination of micronutrients', of everyone in a population who consumes a fortified food, i.e. increase the population's nutrient intake without the need for a conscious dietary behaviour change. This advantage is particularly beneficial because dietary behaviour change is a notoriously difficult outcome to achieve and sustain. Evaluations of social marketing campaigns promoting dietary guideline-type messages consistently indicate that when positive outcomes are identified, they are usually over-represented among the relatively well-off population groups in society, sometimes referred to as the 'worried well'. In comparison, population groups who would most benefit from dietary change may not have the resources or opportunities to act on the campaign's message. This situation highlights the equitable nature of food fortification programmes relative to many alternative policy interventions (assuming those population groups most in need of raised nutrient exposure are able to afford, access, and have available the fortified foods). In addition, food fortification can be introduced relatively quickly and delivered efficiently through increasingly centralized food systems to rapidly raise nutrient exposures for populations. In the context of responding to calls for action on malnutrition, especially undernutrition of various micronutrients, the World Bank has described food fortification as the technology that offers the largest opportunity to improve lives considering its relatively low cost and short time to effect change (24).

Those who are more cautious about food fortification suggest that policy decisions should be made in the context of uncertainties with scientific evidence and ethical considerations. Scientific uncertainties relate to the public health effectiveness of food fortification, as well as its safety implications. According to a former president of the International Union of Nutritional Sciences, food fortification is often misused to be a form of 'technological fix', in which a diversity of different nutrients are used to act on different health problems, resulting in a 'patchwork quilt' effect of interventions. He suggests that greater investment in promoting primary foods would result in a more effective and safer foundation to achieve a balanced healthy diet that consists of many ingredients and interactions that cannot be accommodated by food fortification (25). From an ethical perspective, food fortification raises concerns about the rights of individuals, population groups, and the public as a whole. For example, whereas an advantage of mandatory fortification of a food staple is that it passively exposes a target population to raised levels of a nutrient, its non-selective nature is a double-edged sword, because it does not discriminate and will expose all consumers to a raised level of the nutrient regardless of whether they will gain any benefit from this exposure or not.

It is clear that expectations associated with mandatory food fortification need to be kept in perspective. According to the WHO, whereas food fortification can be a powerful technology for reducing micronutrient malnutrition, it should not be positioned as a stand-alone solution, and instead be regarded as part of an integrated approach to prevent micronutrient malnutrition along with other approaches (26). There are a number of causes of micronutrient malnutrition, not least poverty. Development programmes to tackle poverty may include food fortification programmes. However, often these fortification programmes may be replaced or complemented with targeted activities, such as income generation, nutrient supplementation, dietary diversification, and various public health measures focusing on water sanitation and deworming (27).

Voluntary food fortification raises another set of potential public health concerns. Whereas voluntarily-fortified foods may provide an extra source of nutrients for the population that eats the foods, high consumers of these foods may exceed the upper level of intake for safety for a particular nutrient (28). In addition, many voluntarily-fortified foods contain high levels of sugar and salt, such that at the same time that they are providing extra nutrients, they may be contributing to dietary imbalances. Public health nutritionists question whether the progressive permitting of a wider range of fortified foods, with accompanying marketing claims, creates consumer confusion about what constitutes a healthy and balanced diet. For example, does the wider availability and marketing of calcium-fortified fruit drinks lead to their substitution for milk?

The contested nature of food fortification provides fertile territory for competing views in policy debates, such as determining the relative degree of control the state and the market should have over the regulation of food fortification.

For example, the following two statements typify the two extremes of the arguments around fortification:

1 We have evolved eating large amounts of fruit and vegetables obtained from local food systems—we should encourage people to eat more locally-produced fruit and vegetables and discourage the widespread fortification of highly processed foods.

or

2 It is idealistic to expect people to eat more fruit and vegetables—with food science and global food system capabilities, we should just let popular fast food and soft drink companies add more nutrients to their food products so long as it doesn't cause harm.

The existence of demonstrated benefits alongside contested evidence, ethics, and political dimensions to the food fortification–public health relationship highlights that it would be naïve to conclude that the current proliferation of fortified foods is definitively good or bad for public health. Worryingly, although there are these many public health concerns, there is a lack of monitoring and evaluation of the public health implications of food fortification. For instance, it has been noted that rarely has the effectiveness of food fortification programmes been properly evaluated for their impact on nutritional status (26). Greater investment in monitoring and evaluation of food fortification programmes is indicated, but is of itself not sufficient to understand the public health considerations. Investigations that critically analyse the public health benefits, risks, and ethical considerations of food fortification policies, and contribute to understanding how and why they are being made, are needed to help strengthen food fortification's capacity to protect and promote public health into the future.

The research aim

In spite of the significant impact of food fortification policy on the food supply and public health, public health practitioners often have limited opportunity and awareness to participate in food fortification policy development. Therefore, if practitioners want to influence food fortification activities, an essential prerequisite is to gain an understanding of the issues and policy-making so they have a greater capacity to participate in the policy process, to have their voice heard, and to influence decisions (29). In this regard, the research aim of this investigation was to provide insights into the public health benefits, risks, and ethical considerations of food fortification and understandings of its policy-making processes. It is intended that the achievement of this research aim will help students and practitioners identify how food fortification policy processes and subsequent policy outcomes might be improved to further protect and promote public health.

This investigation was informed by a policy science perspective. Policy science is concerned with identifying and analysing the political variables (determinants) of policies as well as articulating the mechanisms, processes, and structures through which these variables are expressed and exert their influence over policy-making (30). In particular, the findings and lessons from this investigation emerged from a critical analysis of food fortification policy. This critical analysis approach meant not passively accepting claims about policy-making on face value, and instead striving to uncover information to help assess the implications of food fortification policies, and to analyse how and why such policies are made. The critical analysis was not about setting up food fortification policy for criticism. Rather it was a strategic acknowledgement of the political realities of policy-making that need to be made clear from the outset, so that a meaningful investigation can then be undertaken and insights gained to contribute to a constructive outcome.

A policy science perspective challenges the assumption that scientific facts exist as value-free entities that are simply waiting to be discovered by researchers so as to provide inputs to incrementally expand the knowledge base for food fortification. Policy science posits that, although the intention is that food fortification policy be the product of rational processes informed by evidence and ethical reasoning systems, it is inevitable that these rational processes are subject to influences by actors, activities, and agendas that shape how they are constructed, interpreted, and applied. For instance, the way that a research investigation is prioritized and a question is framed is a human judgement and determines what facts are (and are not) able to be collected. Similarly, human judgement is required to complement the available evidence and ethical considerations to weigh up uncertainties, assumptions and the pros and cons of different health policy interventions (31). It is the presence of human judgements in research and policy processes that has led policy scientists to emphasize the explanatory role of values, beliefs, and interests in influencing the use of evidence in health policy-making (32). As Parsons comments:

> A problem has to be defined, structured, located within certain boundaries and be given a name. How this process happens proves crucial for the way in which a policy is addressed to a given problem. The words and concepts we employ to describe, analyse or categorize a problem will frame and mould the reality to which we seek to apply a policy or 'solution'. The fact that we may share the same data, or at least believe that we share the same data, does not mean that we shall see the same thing. Values, beliefs, ideologies, interests and bias all shape perceptions of reality (33, p. 88).

Following this assessment it becomes clear that if facts are value-laden then by extension the translation of knowledge into evidence-based guidelines and public policy cannot be a 'politically neutral exercise' (34). It is this logic that led this investigation to challenge assumptions that there exists a rational and linear relationship between evidence and policy outcomes. Instead it viewed the use of evidence and ethics in policy-making as being inherently political.

The research questions asked of the investigation were:

1 What are the public health benefits, risks, and ethical considerations associated with food fortification?

2 How and why are food fortification policies made?

This is a novel orientation for food fortification research, because the focus of the investigation is on generating evidence *of* the food fortification policy process with the intention of informing food fortification policies and practices in general. It is distinct from conventional epidemiological and evaluation studies, where the focus is on generating evidence that can be used *for* designing or amending individual food fortification programmes.

How the research was organized

An innovative approach in organizing the research to answer the research questions was required, because food fortification policy is a complex and broad topic to investigate. The sheer size and complexity of this form of technological intervention meant that it presented strategic and practical research challenges. From a strategic perspective, standard lines of inquiry that attempt to assess the impact of food fortification and analyse how and why it was made might be limited, because it has many different facets and applications. It was not the intention in a book of this type to undertake a comprehensive assessment and analysis of food fortification, nor to provide definitive answers on the topic. Instead, this book takes a novel path in providing some rational insights and reasoned findings to the aforementioned guiding research questions on food fortification policy in general, speculation on the direction food fortification is headed, and suggestions for progressing food fortification policy and practice into the future.

The frame of reference for the investigation was food fortification as a technological intervention for public health nutrition policy. It is to food fortification (and its policy processes) in total that the investigation's findings are generalized. This is in contrast to an investigation where the frame of reference is a nutrition problem and how food fortification might help solve this problem. Findings from this second frame of reference cannot be generalized to inform food fortification policy in total. Having stated that, rather than attempting to tackle food fortification as one coherent whole, the research underpinning this investigation was based on positioning food fortification as a broad technological intervention that comprised a number of different types. In order to understand the topic in its entirety, it was pulled apart into individual interventions, or case studies, that were more manageable and able to be interrogated thoroughly. The findings from these individual case studies were then collated and interpreted to inform a picture of what was happening with food fortification as a whole.

This research approach presented a practical problem. There are many different food fortification interventions underway, tackling many different policy problems, in a variety of circumstances. The challenge was to comprehensively and systematically capture what was happening and be able to present the whole as being representative. In addition, the policy problems that food fortification seeks to address, such as micronutrient malnutrition, are often classic examples of so-called 'wicked' problems in public policy (35). They are wicked problems because they can be open-ended and intractable, involve contested policy 'solutions', and regularly challenge the assumption that, so long as there is sufficient evidence available, rational policy planning and implementation will follow (36).

These challenges meant that, to achieve the book's purpose, the investigation needed to extend beyond an analysis of an indeterminate number of randomly selected individual case studies, to enable a rigorous and in-depth analysis of food fortification as a whole. Therefore, a conceptual framework was developed to sample and then assess and analyse case studies in a way that was both strategically meaningful and manageable. The conceptual framework is based on the premise that not all food fortification policies and interventions are the same. The problems and circumstances associated with food fortification are varied, as is the case for food fortification.

The investigation's conceptual framework details plausible public health rationales for undertaking mandatory food fortification. It draws on the following Codex condition that should be fulfilled for any fortification programme:

> There should be a demonstrated need for increasing the intake of an essential nutrient in one or more population groups. This may be in the form of actual clinical or subclinical evidence of deficiency, estimates indicating low levels of intake of nutrients or possible deficiencies likely to develop because of changes taking place in food habits (5, p. 3).

Consistent with this condition, there are three plausible public health rationales for increasing the intake of an essential nutrient in one or more population groups:

1 The food supply is unable to provide sufficient nutrients.

2 The presence of a peculiar physiological condition in certain individuals resulting in a raised nutrient requirement for those individuals.

3 A reduction in exposure to the primary source of a nutrient.

For the purposes of the present investigation, each of these public health rationales for food fortification was linked with a policy problem for which there are one or more underlying causes as outlined in the conceptual framework. Following this outlining of the problem causation, the conceptual framework then lists the multiple potential policy solutions available for each policy problem. A mandatory food fortification case study for each public health rationale was selected (Chapters 5–7). Each case study was assessed for its public health benefits, risks, and ethical considerations in preventing and controlling the policy problem associated with each rationale in absolute terms as well as relative to other potential policy solutions. The findings from each assessment then provided a basis against which the findings of the subsequent analysis of how and why the case study was made could be compared.

This conceptual framework is outlined in Table 1.1 and includes the representative case studies.

How the book is structured

This book is structured into three sections:

Section 1: The evidential, ethical, and political underpinnings of food fortification

This section provides the foundation for undertaking the book's investigation, as detailed in Chapters 2–4. It explains the evidence and ethical and political perspectives around food fortification that underpin the investigation and that gave the book its title, as well as outlining the case study research design and methods that shaped the investigation.

Chapter 2 describes the role of evidence and ethics in informing food fortification policy-making and is illustrated with the current international approaches to putting these into practice. Also is presented is a review of theories and models of evidence- and ethics-informed practice that provided theory-driven insights for guiding the research and a basis for comparing observations.

Chapter 3 details the actors, activities, and agendas that influence how and why evidence and ethics inform food fortification policy-making.

Chapter 4 presents the case study research design and methods that were undertaken for this investigation.

Section 2: The case studies

Following the three foundation chapters of Section 1, the second section of the book presents three topical case studies:

Chapter 5, Case study 1: universal salt iodization as an intervention to help prevent iodine deficiency disorders.

Table 1.1 Conceptual framework for organizing the book's investigation into mandatory food fortification policy

Public health rationale for increasing the intake of a nutrient	The policy 'problem'	Underlying causes of the policy problem	Potential policy 'solutions'	The mandatory food fortification case study for the public health rationale
(1) The food supply is unable to provide sufficient nutrients	Micronutrient malnutrition	Inherent nutrient deficiency in the food supply Poverty and food insecurity (e.g. poor food availability, affordability, and accessibility) Presence of inhibitory dietary components (e.g. phytates binding iron and zinc, non-detoxified cassava and iodine)	Mandatory food fortification Voluntary food fortification Supplementation Public health, social, and/or agricultural development measures Nutrition education Maintaining the status quo	Universal salt iodization to help prevent iodine deficiency disorders (Chapter 4)
(2) Certain individuals have nutrient requirements higher than reference standards[a]	Neural tube defects	Primarily thought to be genetic polymorphisms affecting nutrient metabolism in certain at-risk individuals in combination with environmental influences	Mandatory food fortification Voluntary food fortification Supplementation Nutrition education Maintaining the status quo	Mandatory flour fortification with folic acid to help reduce the risk of neural tube defects (Chapter 6)[a]

| (3) There is a reduction in exposure to the primary source of a nutrient | Vitamin D deficiency | Living conditions

Cultural, religious, and social customs

Concern about risks associated with exposure to the primary source | Mandatory food fortification

Voluntary food fortification

Public health measures—promoting safe sunlight exposure

Supplementation

Nutrition education

Maintaining the status quo | Mandatory milk fortification with vitamin D to help prevent vitamin D deficiency (Chapter 7) |

[a]This public health rationale is associated with a secondary policy problem—micronutrient malnutrition, when its underlying causation is the presence of a parasite infection or a related medical condition affecting nutrient absorption, metabolism, and/or blood, urine, faeces loss. In this circumstance, affected individuals have a nutrient intake requirement higher than reference standards to compensate for the impact of their health condition. The policy problem is not a consequence of an inherent physiological condition influencing a nutrient requirement. Potential policy solutions consistent with those listed to help prevent neural tube defects are relevant for this particular policy problem. In addition, the policy solution of public health, social, and/or agricultural development measures is indicated.

Chapter 6, Case study 2: mandatory flour fortification with folic acid to help reduce the risk of neural tube defects.

Chapter 7, Case study 3: mandatory milk fortification with vitamin D to help prevent vitamin D deficiency.

Each case study was selected as being representative of one of the three plausible public health rationales for food fortification (see Table 1.1). The reasoning behind the selection process is described in Chapters 5–7. Collectively, this second section of the book illustrates a research approach that is based on a single case-study design applied three times, so that all three of the identified public health rationales for food fortification policy are addressed. For each individual case study, the evidence-informed public health benefits and risks, as well as ethical considerations, are assessed and compared with policy alternatives and the policy-making process is critically analysed.

Section 3: Insights from the past and present, and a view to the future

In the book's third and final section, the collective findings from all three case studies are analysed, insights that emerge are discussed, and learnings are identified.

Chapter 8 discusses what the book's investigation reveals about the interplay between evidence, ethics, and politics when using food fortification as a technology to protect and promote public health.

Chapter 9 discusses the likely direction food fortification is headed and provides suggested priority activities to progress food fortification policy and practice into the future.

Chapter 10 provides the book's conclusion and presents the lessons learned from the investigation in relation to what the findings might mean for food fortification policy and practice.

References

1. World Health Organization and Office of the United Nations High Commissioner for Human Rights. *Fact sheet: the right to health*. Geneva: WHO and Office of the UN High Commissioner for Human Rights; 2007 [cited 12 January 2012]. Available from: http://www.who.int/mediacentre/factsheets/fs323_en.pdf.

2. Eaton S, Eaton Sr, Konner M, Shostak M. An evolutionary perspective enhances understanding of human nutritional requirements. *Journal of Nutrition* 1996; 126(6):1732–40.

3. Wells S. *Pandora's seed: why the hunter-gatherer holds the key to our survival*. London: Penguin UK; 2011.

4. Codex Alimentarius Commission. Report of the thirty third session of the Codex Committee on nutrition and foods for special dietary uses. Bad Soden am Taunus, Germany; 14–18 November 2011.

5. Codex Alimentarius Commission. *General principles for the addition of essential nutrients to foods (CAC/GL 09-1987, amended 1989, 1991)*; 1987 [cited 20 September 2012]. Available from: http://www.codexalimentarius.org/standards/list-of-standards/en/.

6. Mejia L. Fortification of foods: historical development and current practices. *Food and Nutrition Bulletin* 1994; 15(4):278-1.

7. Burgi H, Supersaxo Z, Selz B. Iodine deficiency diseases in Switzerland one hundred years after Theodor Kocher's survey: a historical review with some new goitre prevalence data. *Acta Endocrinologica (Copenhagen)* 1990; 123(6):577–90.

8. Zimmermann M. Research on iodine deficiency and goiter in the 19th and early 20th centuries. *Journal of Nutrition* 2008; 138(11):2060–3.

9. United Nations System Standing Committee on Nutrition. *Sixth report on the world nutrition situation*. Geneva: UNSCN; 2010 [cited 26 February 2012]. Available from: http://www.unscn.org/files/Publications/RWNS6/html/index.html.

10. Black R, Allen L, Bhutta Z, Caulfield L, de Onis M, Ezzati M, *et al.* Maternal and child undernutrition: global and regional exposures and health consequences. *Lancet* 2008; 371:243–60.

11. World Health Organization. *WHA45.33 National strategies for prevention and control of micronutrient malnutrition, Geneva, 4–14 May* Geneva: WHO; 1992 [cited 11 August 2011]. Available from: http://www.who.int/nutrition/topics/wha_nutrition_mnm/en/index.html.

12. United Nations International Children's Emergency Fund. *The state of the world's children. Special edition. Celebrating 20 years of the Convention on the Rights of the Child.* New York: UNICEF; 2009 [cited September 2011]. Available from: www.unicef.org/rightsite/sowc/pdfs/SOWC_Spec%20Ed_CRC_Main%20Report_EN_090409.pdf.

13. United Nations System Standing Committee on Nutrition. *Scaling Up Nutrition: A Framework for Action.* Based on a series of consultations hosted by the Center for Global Development, the International Conference on Nutrition, USAID, UNICEF and the World Bank; 2010.

14. US Department of Agriculture ERC. *Global food markets: global food industry structure.* Washington, DC: USDA; 2011 [cited July 2011]. Available from: http://www.ers.usda.gov/Briefing/GlobalFoodMarkets/Industry.htm.

15. http://www.pourontheprofits.com [cited 29 November 2011]. Available from: http://www.pourontheprofits.com.

16. Centers for Disease Control and Prevention. Trends in wheat flour fortification with folic acid and iron—worldwide, 2004 and 2007. *Morbidity and Mortality Weekly Report Recommendation Report* 2008; 57:8–10.

17. Flour Fortification Initiative. *Public-private-civic investment in each nation.* [cited 19 March 2012]. Available from: http://www.sph.emory.edu/wheatflour/index.php.

18. Flynn A, Hirvonen T, Mensink G, Ocke M, Serra-Majem L, Stos K, *et al.* Intake of selected nutrients from foods, from fortification and from supplements in various European countries. *Food & Nutrition Research Supplement* 1, 2009. DOI: 10.3402/fnr.v53i0.2038.

19. Fulgoni V, Keast D, Bailey R, Dwyer J. Foods, fortificants, and supplements: where do Americans get their nutrients? *Journal of Nutrition* 2011; 141(10):1847–54.

20. International Food Information Council Foundation. *Food and health survey: consumer attitudes toward food safety, nutrition and health, a trended survey,* 5 May 2011.

Washington, DC: International Food Information Council Foundation; 2011 [cited 2 December 2011]. Available from: http://www.foodinsight.org/Content/3840/2011%20IFIC%20FDTN%20Food%20and%20Health%20Survey.pdf.

21. *Food Navigator.* 2011 [cited 2 December 2011]. Available from: http://www.foodnavigator-usa.com/Product-Categories/Health-and-nutritional-ingredients/Fortification-drives-consumer-definition-of-healthy.

22. Global Industry Analysts Inc. Global Vitamins Market to Reach US$3.3 Billion by 2015, According to a New Report by Global Industry Analysts, Inc. *Vocus PRW Holdings, LLC* February 7 2011 [updated February 7 2011; cited 3 December 2011]. Available from: http://www.prweb.com/releases/vitamins/food_supplements/prweb8114929.htm.

23. Jacobs DR, Jr, Mursu J, Meyer KA. The importance of food. *Archives of Pediatrics and Adolescent Medicine* 2012; 166(2):187–8.

24. The World Bank. *Repositioning nutrition as central to development.* Washington, DC: The World Bank; 2006 [cited 27 April 2012]. Available from: http://siteresources.worldbank.org/NUTRITION/Resources/281846-1131636806329/NutritionStrategy.pdf.

25. Wahlqvist M. National food fortification: a dialogue with reference to Asia: policy in evolution. *Asia Pacific Journal of Clinical Nutrition* 2008; 17(Suppl 1):24–9.

26. Allen L, de Benoist B, Dary O, Hurrell R. *Guidelines on food fortification with micronutrients.* Geneva: World Health Organization; 2006 [cited 25 September 2012]. Available from: http://www.who.int/nutrition/publications/guide_food_fortification_micronutrients.pdf.

27. Howson C, Kennedy E, Horwitz A (eds). *Prevention of micronutrient deficiencies: tools for policy makers and public health workers.* Washington, DC: National Academy Press; 1998.

28. Boilson A, Staines A, Kelleher C, Daly L, Shirley I, Shrivastava A, et al. Unmetabolized folic acid prevalence is widespread in the older Irish population despite the lack of a mandatory fortification program. *American Journal of Clinical Nutrition* 2012; 96(3):613–21.

29. Coveney J. Analyzing public health policy: three approaches. *Health Promotion Practice* 2010; 11(4):515–21.

30. Navarro V. Politics and health: a neglected area of research. *European Journal of Public Health* 2008; 18(4):354–5.

31. Oxman A, Lavis J, Fretheim A, Lewin S. SUPPORT tools for evidence-informed health Policymaking (STP) 16: using research evidence in balancing the pros and cons of policies. *Health Research Policy and Systems* 2009; 7(Suppl 1):S16.

32. de Leeuw E. Health policy, epidemiology and power: the interest web. *Health Promotion International* 1993; 8(1):49–52.

33. Parsons W. *Public policy: an introduction to the theory and practice of policy analysis.* Cheltenham: Edward Elgar Publishing Ltd; 1995.

34. Greenhalgh T, Wieringa S. Is it time to drop the 'knowledge translation' metaphor? A critical literature review. *Journal of the Royal Society of Medicine* 2011; 104(12):501–9.

35. Rittel HWJ, Webber MM. Dilemmas in a general theory of planning. *Policy Sciences* 1973; 4(2):155–69.

36. Head B. Wicked problems in public policy. *Public Policy* 2008; 3(2):101–18.

Section 1

The evidential, ethical, and political underpinnings of food fortification

In most countries fortified foods are available in the marketplace by virtue of permissions expressed in food law and regulatory frameworks. Therefore fortified food products cannot appear arbitrarily in the marketplace even if food manufacturers possess the technological capacity to ensure their supply or there exists demand for their availability from various interest groups. There are food laws and regulations that specify whether or not food fortification is permitted and, if so, under what conditions. These conditions include technical details such as which foods can be fortified with which nutrients in what form, at what levels, and with what associated claims. Food law and regulatory frameworks manage food fortification in two distinct orientations. Proactively, they manage food fortification as an intervention to help promote public health. Reactively, they manage food fortification so that the public's health and safety is protected.

In order to assess the public health benefits, risks, and ethical considerations of food fortification activities, and to analyse how and why such activities take place, there is a need to gain a basic understanding of the relationship between food laws and regulations, and food fortification. Providing the information to gain this basic understanding is the purpose of this section of the book. The three chapters collectively describe the evidence, the ethics, and the politics associated with food laws and regulations and which subsequently underpin food fortification. The descriptions provided the information that formed the platform from which this book's investigation was undertaken. In particular, the case study investigations presented in Section 2 drew on this information when conducting their assessments and analyses.

In Chapter 2 the evidential and ethical reasoning systems that inform food fortification policy and practice are presented. These reasoning systems do not talk for themselves. The actors, their activities, and the agendas shaping food regulatory systems within which the reasoning systems operate are described in Chapter 3. The descriptions in these first two chapters highlight the contested nature of food fortification policy-making and practice. Therefore, Chapter 3 also provides a review of major policy science theoretical frameworks as a basis for informing the investigation into the political nature of food fortification activities. In Chapter 4 the method that was used to undertake the research reported in this book is presented.

Chapter 2

Food fortification evidence and ethics

Evidence-informed health policy-making is an approach to policy decisions that aims to ensure that decision making is well-informed by the best available research evidence.

(Reproduced with permission from Oxman A, Lavis J, Fretheim A, Lewin S. SUPPORT tools for evidence-informed health Policymaking (STP) 16: using research evidence in balancing the pros and cons of policies. Health Research Policy and Systems 2009; 7 Suppl 1: S16.(1))

Food fortification is as much about ethics and society as it is about science . . . While traditionally staple foods such as flour, cereals and spreads have been seen as good 'vehicles' for added nutrients . . . the question remains: is mass medication through the food we eat the way to go?

(Reproduced from Ursula Arens, spokeswoman for the British Dietetic Association, as quoted in The Independent, Friday 3 February 2012, page 36, Meg Carter, with permission from The Independent, www.independent.co.uk (2))

Introduction

The 'protection of public health and safety' is typically the primary objective for national and international food regulatory authorities when developing food fortification policy and programmes. Curiously, what this means in practice has not been clearly defined (3). Therefore, its interpretation and application can be uncertain. There are two particular uncertainties that have a bearing on food fortification policy-making. First, what exactly is the meaning ascribed to the word, '*protection*' in the objective 'protection of public health and safety'? Might the objective be applied to assess benefits associated with using mandatory food fortification to protect against a population-wide nutrient deficiency? Alternatively, might the objective be applied to assess potential risks associated with permitting the introduction of a novel voluntarily-fortified food into the marketplace?

A second area of uncertainty relates to the nature and scope of the phrase '*public health and safety*'. Should the phrase be interpreted in terms of a relatively immediate impact at the individual level, or as a longer-term impact at the population level? For example, should the assessment of a proposed food fortification activity be confined to its potential for immediate harm resulting from excessive nutrient intake, or be extended to include broader public health implications such as its potential to foster dietary imbalances.

Food fortification can be a vexed public health topic that creates unusual dilemmas for policy-makers. People can have opposing views about how to regulate food fortification in situations where there is a confluence of competing agendas for this technology, such as those which arise when a public health agenda may clash with a food marketing agenda. Moreover, food fortification exposes everyone who consumes the fortified food to a raised level of one or more fortificants. This exposure has ethical consequences as it can (though not always) create conflicts between the freedoms and needs of the individual and the freedoms and needs of the population. How can policy-makers resolve these dilemmas, especially if there are alternative policy interventions available, and against which food fortification might be compared? One approach is to rely on opinion and speculation. A more commonly accepted approach is to apply systems of reasoning to inform food fortification policy and programmes.

In the absence of a clear definition of the objective of protecting public health and safety, meaning is acquired through the use of evidence and ethics in food fortification policy-making. Evidence and ethics provide systems of reasoning that aim to protect public health and safety in food fortification policies and programmes via the application of explicit evaluative frameworks. The purpose of this chapter is to provide a critical description of these evidential and ethical evaluative frameworks. The first section outlines two perspectives for applying evidential evaluative frameworks in a food fortification context: evidence-informed policy for using food fortification as a technological intervention to *promote* public health, and an evidence-informed nutritional risk analysis framework to *protect* public health in response to food fortification proposals. The next section provides an outline of ethical considerations in food fortification and is followed by a review of how the more prominent ethical theories and principles can be applied to help assess policy responses. In the final section, a review of theories and models of evidence- and ethics-informed public health policy-making is presented.

Food fortification evidence

It is a broadly accepted principle that food fortification policy and programmes should be informed by scientific evidence. This acceptance resides within the fundamental epistemological notion about the role of knowledge as a guide for human action. A core appeal of evidence-informed policy-making is that it points to objectivity in justifying decisions (4).

What is less well accepted is what constitutes the evidence that should be used to inform food fortification policy and programme decision-making. When evaluating the benefits and risks of food fortification interventions (and alternative policy interventions with which food fortification is compared), researchers and policy-makers may have a diversity of views. These include: which research questions should be asked and how should they be framed, the scope of the study and how it might be designed, and which methods are used. Which views prevail determines what evidence 'counts'.

This section provides a description of the current orthodoxy for using evidence to inform food fortification policy-making and programmes from two perspectives, using food fortification to *promote* public health, and *protect* public health, in response to food fortification proposals. The description of each begins with an overview of the purpose of evidence-informed practice and the different viewpoints regarding what constitutes evidence for policy-making. Typically, national food regulatory authorities have established procedures specifying the way that evidence is to be collected, assessed, and synthesized to inform food fortification policy-making. It is not feasible to present a comprehensive description of the array of national procedures for food fortification evidence-informed practice. Instead, the procedures that have been established by United Nation (UN) agencies (and adopted by many national authorities) are outlined here as exemplars for such processes. These UN procedures provide a template for practice in many countries.

Evidence-informed policy when using food fortification to *promote* public health

What is the purpose of evidence-informed policy and practice in this promotion perspective?

In this perspective, evidence is used primarily to inform policy-makers about the public health benefits of a food fortification intervention itself and in comparison with alternative interventions. Evidence may be obtained from the evaluation of the effectiveness of existing interventions or by assessing the efficacy of the various interventions using experimental or non-experimental studies.

What constitutes evidence in this promotion perspective?

The conventional view of what constitutes evidence to inform policy-making in this perspective is that the higher the quality of the evidence, the better. This view has been carried over from the evidence-based medicine (EBM) movement. EBM has been defined as: 'The conscientious, explicit, and judicious use of current best evidence in making decisions about the care of individual patients' (5). The EBM movement evolved from the work of pioneers such as English physician Archie Cochrane, who observed and then expressed concern about the number of clinical care decisions that were informed by intuition and opinion rather than high quality evidence (6).

Critical procedures have been established to facilitate EBM and the extrapolation of its principles to decision-making for health policy settings. The quality of evidence is judged by ranking it according to an evidence hierarchy. The hierarchy is based on the ability of the research method, from which the evidence is derived, to control for bias when investigating relationships. For instance, evidence derived from experimental research methods such as randomized controlled trials (RCTs) is considered high quality, because such trials are able to establish internal validity (7). Internal validity is the validity with which it can be inferred that a relationship between two variables is causal (or the absence of a relationship implies the absence of cause) (8). It is the ability of experimental research methods to reduce relationships to specific inputs and outcomes and remove potential confounding factors that is critical in establishing internal validity. This characteristic of experimental research methods of tightly framing the relationship under investigation is a 'reductionist' approach. In nutrition, complying with procedures that support a reductionist approach requires dissecting complex food and health relationships into constituent parts to isolate precise linear relationships between a specific food component, such as a nutrient, and a specific metabolic pathway (9).

A number of public health nutritionists question the suitability of the reductionist underpinnings to the current evidence hierarchy approach to assess the quality of evidence available to inform nutrition-related policies including food fortification. As Chung comments:

> Whereas the concepts and methods of evidence-based medicine can be applied to nutrition questions, there are important differences between evaluations of drug therapies and nutrient-related health outcomes (10, p. 1099).

Strict adherence to the evidence hierarchy approach can be a problematic basis for appraising evidence to inform nutrition-related policies intended to promote and protect public health from both a technical and a conceptual perspective. From a technical perspective, nutrient interventions generally do not behave in the same way as health care/drug interventions, because they can result in multiple outcomes which may be subtle and take extended periods of time to manifest. In these circumstances, the use of RCTs as a research method is rendered impractical and possibly unethical (11, 12).

In addition to the technical limitations of using RCTs to investigate nutrition relationships is the conceptual limitation that relates to the truism that: 'People eat food, not single food components in isolation'. Reducing the analysis of complex food and health relationships to a series of individual nutrient–metabolic relationships ignores the critical factor that food is a matrix containing a mixture of nutrients that interact synergistically in ways that affect their influence on health outcomes (13). For example, within a food matrix, a single nutrient's bioavailability might be increased or reduced in response to the presence of other nutrients and food components. Within a food matrix a nutrient will likely influence metabolic pathways in different ways to those identified from investigating the nutrient in isolation (14). Beyond the complexity of food–metabolic relationships is the increasing recognition of the importance of dietary patterns in influencing health outcomes. For example, the Mediterranean diet is now recognized as being of world heritage significance (15) and comprises a combination of foods that contribute to a number of biological, health, cultural, environmental, and social benefits (16).

Moreover, the causes of inadequate nutrient intakes can be found in a variety of social, economic, environmental, and health circumstances (see Chapter 1). Interventions such as those that support poverty alleviation programmes, invest in agricultural development, or promote healthy dietary behaviours, might be indicated to directly address these causes. A variety of methods are required to evaluate the relative benefits of these different policy interventions in mitigating the causes and thereby helping achieve adequate nutrient intakes. Observational studies (cohort studies and case–control studies) are well suited to investigating such interventions and consequently have high external validity, i.e. the validity with which it can be inferred that a presumed causal relationship can be generalized to real-world settings (8).

Investigating interactions within complex systems, whether between food and health, traditional cuisines and multiple health outcomes, or social/environmental/public health interventions and nutrient intake patterns, is the antithesis of a reductionist approach. It is by maintaining the integrity of the complex interactions that observational study designs are able to extrapolate patterns of interaction. Conversely, the reductionist approach of experimental study designs attempts to control and organize any interactions into a collection of precise individual linear relationships, externalizing the very factors that help explain the interactions. Inevitably, there is a trade-off between internal and external validity in using different study designs to provide evidence to inform decision-making for policies and programmes to address inadequate nutrient intakes. As the rigour of the study design to generate efficacy evidence increases, the generalizability and relevance of extrapolating the research evidence to infer a public health benefit tend to diminish.

The contemporary exemplar in this promotion perspective

In 2007, following a call from the 58th World Health Assembly (WHA), the World Health Organization (WHO) director general established the guidelines review committee. Its purpose was to develop and implement procedures to ensure that WHO guidelines are developed in ways consistent with best practice, emphasizing the appropriate use of evidence. In 2009, the process for developing evidence-informed guidelines was formalized when the WHO adopted a nine-step procedure outlined in the WHO handbook for guideline development (17) and reproduced in Figure 2.1.

This guideline development process supports a reductionist approach to investigating nutrition relationships and assessing the quality of evidence. A detailed description of the application of WHO's guideline development process to the development of micronutrient intervention recommendations has been provided elsewhere (18). This description explains that the WHO's Department of Nutrition for Health and Development (NHD) establishes the priorities for micronutrient interventions requiring updates. It undertakes this role in consultation with other international agencies and academia, and by direct requests from countries or via the WHA. The evidence practice component of the guideline development process (steps 4–6) is outlined as follows:

Step 4: formulation of the research question.

The evidence practice component of the guideline development process starts with this step, the formulation of priority research questions and choice of relevant outcomes. A clearly formulated research question and articulated outcomes provide the foundation for an efficient structuring of the search for, and assessment of, information, in the process of preparing food fortification recommendations.

Step 5: evidence retrieval, assessment, and synthesis.

In 2009, the NHD's micronutrients unit commenced a work programme in collaboration with professional teams from around the world to undertake systematic reviews of micronutrient interventions. The aim was to standardize the way the evidence for the effects and safety of micronutrient interventions

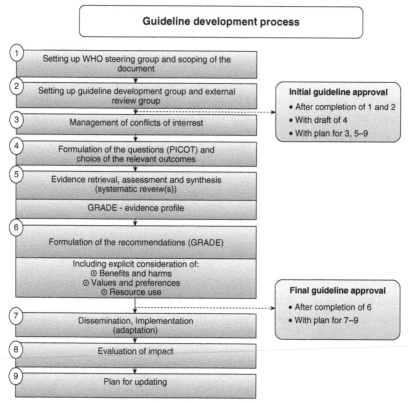

Fig. 2.1 World Health Organization evidence-informed guideline development process.

Reproduced with permission from the World Health Organization Guidelines Review Committee, 2010, World Health Organization guideline development process, figure 4, page 11, Copyright © World Health Organization 2010, available at: http://www.who.int/hiv/topics/mtct/grc_handbook_mar2010_1.pdf.

is summarized, appraised, and synthesized (18). The unit's preference is for systematic reviews that are prepared according to the Cochrane or the Campbell Collaborations' procedures (19). Recognition of the integral collaboration between the WHO and The Cochrane Collaboration was reflected in the WHO awarding The Cochrane Collaboration a seat on the WHA on 24 January 2011 (20).

Systematic reviews involve searching for and collating all the available research on a topic that meets predetermined criteria. The research information is then assessed against guidelines to establish the evidence about an intervention. The reviews are designed to inform the choices that practitioners, consumers, policy-makers, and others face in public health policy by taking into account the benefits, risks, and costs of interventions. The standard protocol for undertaking a systematic review should be prepared in such a way that the procedure is systematic, rigorous, and transparent.

The evidence outputs from a systematic review are not by themselves sufficient to support decision-making. The quality of the evidence also must be taken into account. When preparing evidence summaries for micronutrient interventions, the NHD employs the grading of recommendations assessment, development, and evaluation (GRADE) methodology to assess the overall quality of the evidence (21). The GRADE approach ranks the quality of evidence by considering factors such as the study design from which the evidence was derived. Evidence derived from experimentally designed studies such as RCTs is ranked of higher quality than evidence derived from observational studies such as cohort studies. The reasoning behind this ranking is that the experimental design is better able to remove potential confounders and therefore control for bias when analysing relationships, so that the findings from such studies have a higher internal validity.

Step 6: formulation of recommendations and use of GRADE methodology.

The drafting of WHO food fortification guidelines takes into account both the systematic reviews and the GRADE evidence profiles. The members of the food fortification guideline development group review the evidence and determine the strength of the recommendation by considering benefits and risks of the intervention and factors such as the quality of the available evidence (18).

Challenges in using the evidence hierarchy approach to inform food fortification policy

The GRADE methodology's evidence hierarchy approach is well suited to assess the quality of evidence associated with the potential benefits and risks, and quality of evidence of the efficacy of micronutrient interventions (food fortification and supplementation) under controlled trial conditions. This is because the nutrient(s) with which a food is fortified, or that are distributed as supplementation interventions, and their impact on nutrition outcomes are amenable to a reductionist approach of an experimental study design. However, there are two challenges associated with relying on this approach to appraise evidence which need to be taken into account when such evidence is used to inform food fortification policy-making:

1 The evidence hierarchy creates a non-level playing field for comparing the relative benefits and risks of the available policy interventions for addressing inadequate nutrient intakes

There are a number of policy interventions in addition to micronutrient interventions that are available to help address inadequate nutrient intakes. These include a range of social, environmental, and public health interventions. Whereas experimental research methods are well disposed to evaluate the benefits of single nutrient inputs of fortified food and supplementation interventions, they struggle to accurately portray the evidence associated with relationships in which social, environmental, and public health interventions are being evaluated (22). Different methods are needed to evaluate these non-micronutrient interventions so that the nature and nuances of potential relationships can be accurately captured and evaluated (23). How the evidence provided by different research methods aligned with different interventions is judged predetermines which policy interventions are privileged in decision-making. Non-experimental research methods have lower internal validity than experimental methods and the evidence they provide is ranked as low quality according to the evidence hierarchy approach in decision-making, and is often omitted from the reviews that inform food fortification policy guidelines and recommendations (24). Therefore, those policy interventions that rely on non-experimental research methods to evaluate their impacts are often excluded as recommended policy interventions.

2 Demonstrating food fortification efficacy does not necessarily mean it is effective

The evidence hierarchy approach is well suited to demonstrating the efficacy of food fortification interventions, but this does not necessarily equate to demonstrating their effectiveness or plausibility in a real-world setting (25, 26). For instance, in a controlled trial setting, a food fortification intervention might demonstrate that it can help address a nutrient intake problem, but when scaled up and applied in the real world, if it is not plausibly addressing the underlying cause of the problem, the cause will persist and the problem will require ongoing attention.

Evidence-informed policy when *protecting* public health in response to food fortification proposals

What is the purpose of evidence-informed policy and practice in this protection perspective?

In this perspective, evidence is used to inform policy-makers about the public health risks of a food fortification intervention of itself and relative to the risks associated with alternative interventions. Evidence may be obtained from evaluating the implications of existing interventions or predicting the implications of proposed interventions using dietary modelling procedures.

What constitutes evidence in this protection perspective?

The conventional view of what constitutes evidence to inform policy-making in this perspective has been one derived from research procedures mostly within the discipline of toxicology. In the mid-1990s, the Food and Agriculture Organization (FAO) and WHO developed a risk analysis framework, with the purpose of generating evidence to inform food standards (27). The framework consisted of three inter-related components: risk assessment, risk management, and risk communication. In 2003, the Codex Alimentarius Commission (Codex) adopted the: 'Working principles for risk analysis for application in the framework of the Codex Alimentarius', the objective of which is: 'To provide guidance to the Codex Alimentarius Commission and the joint FAO/WHO expert bodies and consultations so that food safety and health aspects of Codex standards and related texts are based on risk analysis' (28).

These principles have now been adopted in the food regulation work of national regulatory and regional agencies, such as the European Food Safety Agency and UN agencies such as the WHO. They have also been applied to the work of a number of Codex committees, including those working on food additives, contaminants in foods, residues of veterinary drugs in foods, and pesticide residues. In these settings, the risk analysis framework is applied to avoid excessive intakes of potentially toxic food constituents.

However, the applicability of the conventional risk analysis principles to nutrition-related considerations for food is limited. Food is more than just a vehicle for potential risk factors. Primarily, food is a source of nutrients essential for health. Risks associated with the addition of nutrients to foods need to be analysed in relation to both inadequate and excessive intakes. In addition, there may be more chronic nutrition risks associated with food intake. Some foods contain significant amounts of saturated fat, sugar, and salt, and excessive intakes of such foods can result in dietary imbalances and subsequently contribute to chronic diseases such as cardiovascular disease and cancer. Food regulators increasingly use nutritional epidemiology and sophisticated dietary modelling techniques to undertake risk analysis in a nutrition context (29).

The contemporary exemplar in this protection perspective

In 2009, nutritional risk analysis principles were established to guide Codex and its subsidiary bodies in applying nutritional risk analysis to their work. These principles were adapted from the 2003 Codex working principles for risk analysis. The scope of the nutritional risk analysis is to consider the risk of adverse health effects from not just excessive, but also inadequate, nutrient intakes, and the predicted reduction in risk or increase in benefit, respectively, from proposed management strategies (28). In parallel with this extension in scope, there has been an extension of the discipline base for generating evidence so as to include epidemiology and nutrition in the risk assessment step.

These are now being proposed to be taken into account in the review of the Codex principles for the addition of essential nutrients to food (30).

The purpose of nutritional risk analysis is to assess the extent of a nutritional risk, how it might be managed and communicated. Thereby it helps inform whether a risk is acceptable and a food fortification activity might proceed. The three dimensions of the nutritional risk analysis process have been adapted from the working principles for risk analysis for application in the framework of Codex, with the addition of an initial problem formulation stage. A nutritional risk is defined by Codex as being a: 'Function of the probability of an adverse health effect associated with inadequate or excessive intake of a nutrient or related substance and the severity of that effect, consequential to a nutrient-related hazard(s) in food' (31).

The components of the nutritional risk analysis framework are described in the 20th edition of the Codex Alimentarius Commission Procedural Manual (31), from which they are summarized as follows and represented in Figure 2.2.

Nutritional problem formulation stage

The nutritional problem formulation stage is a preliminary risk management activity and establishes the purpose of a nutritional risk assessment and the questions that need to be answered. In the context of analysing possible risk associated with a food fortification programme, the risk may relate to an inadequate intake of a nutrient, an excessive intake of a nutrient, or both, especially when risk is analysed across multiple population groups. Nutritional problems

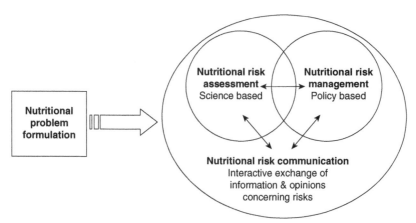

Fig. 2.2 Nutritional risk analysis framework.

Adapted with permission from the World Health Organization, available at http://www.who.int/foodsafety/micro/riskanalysis/en/.

associated with these risks may give rise to the following questions: 'What is the current nutrient intake distribution across the population?' and 'How will different food fortification scenarios affect dietary intake distributions?'. In so doing, the nutritional problem formulation helps identify who should be involved in the nutritional risk assessment, nutritional risk management, and nutritional risk communication processes. It also helps identify how the steps can be coordinated so that the information provided by the risk assessment component can best support the nutritional risk management decision.

Nutritional risk assessment stage

The nutritional risk assessment component incorporates a scientifically-based process for forecasting the impact of possible responses to the food fortification regulations on public health and safety. It is undertaken by relevant scientists and progresses from identifying the nutrient of interest, describing its effect on health, and assessing whether there is a risk (or benefit) to the population, as based on dietary intake (exposure) estimates.

A food regulatory agency applies risk assessment to describe the estimated dietary exposure and to forecast future possible population exposures following scenarios associated with varying the food fortification conditions—depending on what foods and what nutrient levels.

Nutritional risk assessment consists of the following subcomponents: (1) hazard identification, (2) hazard characterization, (3) intake (exposure) assessment, and (4) risk characterization. A brief description of these four subcomponents and how they apply to a food fortification context follows:

1 Hazard identification: is the effect resulting from either risk of too high a nutrient intake and subsequent adverse effects, or risk of too low a nutrient intake and subsequent adverse effects of risk of inadequacy or deficiency. It includes the identification of hazardous health effects and the corresponding population at risk for the micronutrient of interest.

2 Hazard characterization: describes the dose–response relationship for symptoms of deficiency or excess and adverse effects. Its purpose is to estimate the dose at which the effect takes place. The FAO/WHO have published globally applicable nutrient reference standards for both average nutrient requirements for adequacy and upper levels of nutrient intake for excess (32).

3 Intake (exposure) assessment: the population intake needs to be described because the extent of the population risk is characterized by the intake distribution compared with the dose–response characteristics of the hazard. The exposure assessment considers what is known about the distribution of the present habitual nutrient intake at the median and 95th percentile.

The scientific technique of dietary modelling is used to estimate dietary intakes across the population based on the establishment of relevant intake scenarios. The scenarios usually include a reference scenario (e.g. intake based on the current situation) and some relevant simulated scenarios (e.g. micronutrient intake following the introduction of a new fortified food). For each scenario, the habitual intake distribution at a population level is estimated for the micronutrient of interest.

4 Risk characterization: involves a comparison of intake to nutrient reference standards. Risk characterization results when the information from hazard characterization and intake assessment steps are combined to provide an assessment of the proportion of the population or population subgroups whose habitual intakes exceed or fail to achieve the nutrient reference standards.

Nutritional risk management stage

The nutritional risk management post-risk assessment involves the process of weighing policy alternatives in response to the problem, taking into account the risk assessment and other factors, and selecting options to prevent, reduce, or eliminate the risk to protect public health. Whereas risk assessors might identify a certain proportion of the population exceeding the upper level of safety for a nutrient, risk managers must decide if this is a problem, and if so, what should be done about it. Risk management options related to food fortification might include determining: whether the fortification should be mandatory or voluntary, which foods are eligible for fortification, the level of nutrient addition permitted, the suitability of foods that contain high levels of fat, sugar and salt, and labelling advice to accompany the fortification. It is important for the integrity of the overall risk analysis process that the decision-makers who undertake the risk management step (in consultation with interested parties) are distinct from the scientists who undertake the risk assessment step. They may be located in different agencies.

Decision-making during the risk management component invariably requires judgements to be made in determining proportionate action in response to risks and benefits assessed in the risk assessment component and consideration of other factors. A further demand on such judgements is the frequent need to make decisions in the face of scientific uncertainty, as acknowledged by the UK Food Standards Agency (FSA) when commenting on the features of the evidence base in regulatory decision-making:

> Often, the evidence underpinning any decision will be incomplete . . . when scientific uncertainty is established, we are open about the uncertainty, and do not allow the absence of certainty to delay us from taking proportionate action (33).

Nutritional risk communication stage

Nutritional risk communication is the interactive and ongoing exchange of information and opinions during the risk assessment and risk management components. It is concerned with communicating among risk assessors, risk managers, the public, industry, the academic community, and other interested parties:

1 awareness and understanding of the specific issues under consideration during the risk analysis

2 consistency and transparency in formulating risk management options/recommendations, and

3 a sound basis for understanding the risk management decisions proposed.

The initial problem formulation stage and the inter-relationships among the subsequent three components are presented in Figure 2.2.

Challenges in using the nutritional risk analysis framework to inform food fortification policy

All components of the risk analysis framework are open to interpretation, and as such their application when informing food fortification policy relies on human judgement. For example, there is debate about what constitutes evidence in a nutritional risk analysis framework, with views varying markedly depending on the scope with which risk is interpreted, and the nutritional epidemiology and dietary exposure estimates that are employed in the nutritional risk assessment component. Some approaches adopt a narrow interpretation to the scope of nutritional risk assessment. For example, a project funded by the 'Addition of nutrients to food task force' of the European Branch of the Life Sciences Institute (with members drawn from fortified food manufacturers and a vitamin provider) proposed a dietary modelling technique to estimate the levels of micronutrients that can be added to food without exceeding tolerable upper intakes (34). Other approaches propose models that extend the scope of risk assessment to consider not just immediate risks associated with nutrients exceeding upper safe levels, but also the chronic risks associated with dietary imbalances that may result from the liberal fortification and subsequent marketing of food products high in sugar, fat, and salt (35).

Food fortification ethics

Ethics is a branch of philosophy that deals with the moral consequences of human actions, including public policy interventions. Public health ethics is a nascent field that has emerged from medical ethics (moral considerations associated with patient–doctor interactions) and bioethics (ethical implications of biotechnology), and is concerned with providing moral guidance when planning policy interventions that are intended to have a health benefit for the public (36). A common ethical consequence (though not necessarily always) that arises with public health policy interventions is the conflict between acting for the common good and imposing on individual rights and interfering with personal freedoms. Should the rights and needs of the population take precedence over the rights and needs of the individual, or vice versa?

Food fortification interventions are associated with a number of peculiar ethical conflicts. Mandatory food fortification is highly coercive. Its intention is to deliberately and passively expose all individuals in a population who consume the fortified food to a raised level of the nutrient in the food, thereby encroaching on individuals' personal freedoms. This ethical conflict is exacerbated if the intervention has little benefit and possible harm for certain individuals or groups within the population. An individual may choose to not consume the fortified food, though this usually is impractical as it is typically staple foods that are mandated for fortification, and often such interventions proceed without overt notification to individuals. In these circumstances, policy-makers are confronted with having to make a trade-off between protecting and promoting the health of populations and avoiding imposing on individuals' rights and freedoms.

Voluntary food fortification is less coercive than mandatory food fortification. An individual has a choice to consume the fortified food, its non-fortified equivalent, or neither, as this form of intervention often does not involve staple foods. Nevertheless, it is associated with its own ethical conflicts. Because voluntary food fortification is an intervention that usually is undertaken to achieve commercial objectives, it is implemented in conjunction with marketing claims about health benefits associated with the raised level of a nutrient(s) in the food product. On the one hand, the claims make the presence of the raised nutrient level explicit to an individual. On the other hand, the claims may represent a form of soft coercion if an individual is enticed into believing that they need to consume the food product to protect and promote their health—even when this is not the case. Similarly, it may be technically correct for a food manufacturer to claim that their product is a rich source of an added nutrient, but is it morally correct to make this claim implying that the product is healthy if the product also contains significant amounts of sugar and salt?

Faced with these common ethical conflicts, the main questions for policy-makers are: 'Ought we proceed with a food fortification intervention?', and if so, 'On what grounds and under what conditions?', and if not, 'Why not?'. Further complicating decision-making is the need to weigh up the ethical consequences of food fortification interventions against consequences associated with alternative policy interventions that may offer potential solutions to a policy problem. Alternative policy interventions that are intended to increase the population's exposure to a nutrient(s), such as social marketing campaigns, may be less coercive and have less impact on an individual's liberty, but usually they also are less effective in raising nutrient exposure. Policy-makers cannot just guess how to deal with these conflicts and evidence frameworks cannot provide relevant guidance. Rather, public health ethics can provide moral guidance for addressing such conflicts and pointing to what is required for human well-being (37).

Moral guidance when dealing with the ethical consequences of public health policy interventions logically starts with specifying the pertinent ethical conflicts. The ethical conflicts arising from a public health policy intervention are highly nuanced and depend on the policy problem and the circumstances within which it arises. Nevertheless, the ethical conflict that is most pertinent when considering public health policy interventions is the conflict between individualism (autonomy) and collectivism (needs of the public as a whole). In ethical terms, autonomy refers to an individual's ability to control the direction of their own life and to be respected for their ability to decide for themselves.

There is no simple formula that public health ethics can call upon to resolve ethical conflicts associated with public health policy interventions. Instead, public health ethics operates within theories that draw from moral and political philosophy about what is the common good and the individual good to help apply moral reasoning to policy decision-making.

Moral philosophy informs consequentialist theories. These focus on the consequences of a given policy decision, in essence, saying that the end justifies the means. For example, the theory of utilitarianism posits that policy interventions are morally justified when they are striving to achieve, 'the greatest good for the greatest number', and the preferred intervention is the one that achieves the maximum benefit for public health. By contrast, moral philosophy also informs non-consequentialist theories. These provide a justification for policy decisions on the basis of them being guided by a set of inherent moral principles regardless of the consequence of the decision. In other words, it is the process rather than the outcome against which the moral basis of a policy option should be judged. An example of this theoretical view is a human rights-based approach to justifying policy decisions.

Theories informed from political philosophy offer an alternative viewpoint. For example, liberalism challenges the justification for food fortification policy decisions on the grounds that they infringe on liberty of action in terms of personal freedoms and the capacity of individuals to make free choices. A liberalism viewpoint towards food fortification would be that such interventions are paternalistic in that they are actions of authorities that restrict individuals' freedoms by attempting to influence their behaviours, allegedly for their own good.

These ethical theories can provide insights for reasoning ethical conflicts and analysing the relative consequences of different policy interventions. Yet, theoretically-informed analyses might identify irreconcilable tensions between individual interests and the common good, and it may be that there are no definitive answers forthcoming. In such circumstances, the theoretical insights can be applied to help inform the critical decision-making criterion: 'What is reasonable?', i.e. what would a reasonable person do?

A 'justificatory' approach that complements the ethical analysis is often used to evaluate and defend the different policy interventions available as a potential solution to a policy problem. The justificatory approach involves a process of moral reasoning that might consider certain principles that the public might reasonably be expected to accept as justifying the intervention. A case for defending a certain policy intervention then would involve demonstrating how closely the intervention adheres to important principles. Because it is often difficult for a case for a particular policy intervention to demonstrate consensus across all principles, the principles may need to be prioritized by being given different weightings in the decision-making process, in accordance with the circumstances of the policy problem under consideration. This prioritization process is informed by insights from ethical theories.

One practical example of the justificatory approach during the policy-making process is that put forward by Childress et al. (38), in which they propose the use of five principles, or what they call 'justificatory conditions': effectiveness, proportionality, necessity, least infringement, and public justification. Applying these conditions can help provide moral guidance in dealing with ethical conflicts when assessing the relative merits of different policy interventions as potential solutions to a policy problem. In the context of those policy interventions that infringe one or more general moral considerations, the intervention might be defended on the basis of its performance against the following conditions adapted from Childress et al.:

1 Effectiveness: how effective will the policy intervention be in protecting and promoting public health?

2 Proportionality: to what extent will the public health benefits outweigh the infringed general moral considerations, i.e. is the policy intervention not only effective but does it also do more good than harm for individuals and the population as a whole? Factors such as the severity and the prevalence of the public health problem being addressed are relevant considerations in measuring performance against this condition.

3 Necessity: to what extent is the policy intervention necessary to realize the public health goal that is sought?

4 Least infringement: how coercive is the public health policy intervention? Public health policy interventions can vary in their degree of coerciveness, and the less coercive they are, the less their moral infringement (39).

5 Public justification: how are people who are likely to be affected by an infringement to a general moral consideration made aware of the infringement, and have it explained and justified? Factors such as a requirement to receive informed consent, the opportunity for affected people to participate in decision-making, and transparency and accountability of decision-making are relevant considerations in measuring performance against this condition.

The collective performance against these conditions can provide the basis for the case to justify the adoption of a particular public health policy intervention in the context of ethical considerations. Ideally all conditions are met, but this is unlikely in practice, and decision-making often requires the overall balancing of each of the different conditions.

Theories and models of evidence- and ethics-informed public health policy-making

The previous sections outlined the evidential and ethical evaluative frameworks within which food fortification policies and practices are managed and coordinated. Core to these frameworks is the orthodoxy of evidence-based policy and ethical analysis to evaluate food fortification (and alternative interventions) as a policy intervention for protecting and promoting public health. It is assumed that so long as the evidence-based guidelines and risk analysis frameworks, as well as the ethical analysis, are observed, rigorous food fortification policies that promote and protect public health will be made. But is this assumption an accurate and sufficient representation of how and why evidence and ethics are applied and food fortification policy is made in practice?

There are a number of theories and models available to help explain and predict the way that evidential and ethical evaluative frameworks inform public health policy-making. Breton and De Leeuw explain that theories of the policy process formulate propositions on the conditions under which certain policy phenomena are observed and impact on policy outcomes (40). A review of these theories and models was an important preliminary step for the qualitative research of the type undertaken in this book's investigation. It provided insights and understandings to help guide the planning of the analytical stage of this investigation, as well as providing a basis against which its observations were compared and interpreted (41).

This section presents a brief review of theories and models that help explain how and why evidence (and to a lesser extent, ethics) is used in policy-making processes. They are organized into three broad groupings: the rationalist perspective, the research utilization movement, and policy science theoretical frameworks.

The rationalist perspective

Historically it was Laswell, one of the pioneers of the policy sciences, who explained the policy-making process using a 'stages' heuristic (42). This heuristic (an experience-based entity for problem solving) is a model that describes policy-making broadly as progressing through a sequence of distinct stages, starting with problem definition and then moving onto the consideration of policy options, decisions on a policy option(s), implementation, and finally evaluation. The expectation has been that so long as evidence of a sufficient quantity and quality was available and policy options were rigorously assessed, governments would have powerful problem-solving capabilities and policy-making would proceed in an orderly and linear manner through each of the stages in the sequence. The straightforward logic of the stages heuristic is appealing and it persists in many policy textbooks, with the internal structure of such books commonly being organized around describing each of the stages.

The model draws on the rationalist assumption that data are systematically collected and then appraised against criteria to generate the most comprehensive and rigorous evidence base to then inform the policy-making process. In parallel with this model, there has been a significant investment in ranking the methods used to generate evidence for their ability to control for bias and for assessing the quality evidence (see GRADE methodology as described earlier in this chapter). There has also been much investment in conducting research to increase the quantity of evidence available for policy development.

The stages heuristic frequently has been criticized as being an overly simplistic explanation of the policy-making process. Can it be assumed that the generation of an ever-increasing quantity and quality of evidence alone will necessarily drive the formulation of ever-improving food fortification policy? The stages model is not a causal theory in the sense that it cannot offer an explanation of how and why evidence is used in progressing public health policy from one stage to another, nor can it be tested on an empirical basis. Essentially, it prescribes the way policy ought to be made rather than reflecting how policy actually is made. What it cannot do, is to help explain the influence of human involvement in policy processes. This is a critical mediating factor in determining how and why evidence and ethical considerations contribute to policy-making. In order to build a theoretical framework for investigating policy-making, there is a need to move beyond such heuristic devices to explanatory theories.

The research utilization movement

Over the past 20 years, there has been a burgeoning research utilization movement that has contributed valuable conceptual, theoretical, and practical explanations of how and why evidence is used in public health policy-making. A common characteristic within these explanations is the existence of 'two communities' involved in translating evidence into food fortification policy. There is the community of researchers who determine what research questions are asked (and not asked), what research methods are used (and not used), and how the collected evidence is analysed, interpreted, and presented. Then there is the community of policy-makers who determine if, when, and in what form the evidence is used to inform policies and practice. The necessary human involvement introduces subjectivity to the idealized notion of an objective basis to evidence-based policy-making. Inevitably, there are judgements to be made about the interpretation and application of evidence to policy-making. For instance, how to make decisions when there are scientific uncertainties associated with the evidence for a policy problem and/or ethical consequences associated with potential policy solutions to these problems. Hence, it is unlikely that a greater quantity and quality of evidence alone will drive improved food fortification policies.

In response to observed limitations with earlier concepts and theories of policy-making, much policy research has been directed towards gaining greater understanding of what works in using research to support evidence-informed policy-making. In landmark research, Weiss proposed seven models of research utilization, ranging from pragmatic to opportunistic reasons to describe the process by which research informs and is applied to policy-making (43). The investigations undertaken by others involved in developing conceptual frameworks and practical guidance in this area have been described with a diversity of terms including: 'research utilization' (44), 'knowledge translation' (45), 'knowledge transfer' (46), and 'research exchange' (47). A common theme of such research is that the lack of evidence translation arises because of the existence of a 'chasm' between science and policy (48). Advice for responding to observed deficiencies in the integration of research into the policy process focuses on the need to build a bridge (over the chasm) between scientists and policy-makers. Practical suggestions include improving communication to help increase the understanding of each other's work and language, developing political champions to promote the evidence translation, making research findings more accessible to policy-makers, and increasing opportunities for greater interaction between policy-makers and researchers (49, 50). A series of articles has been published (1) and a website established (51) with the intention of helping policy-makers engage with the best available research evidence.

Policy science theoretical frameworks

Since the stages heuristic was first proposed by Laswell, the policy science literature has reported hundreds of theories and models to help explain and predict policy processes. It is beyond the scope of this investigation to review all these theories. Instead the present investigation draws on the work of one of the most well-respected policy scientists, Paul Sabatier (52), who has identified several well-validated and consequently more respected policy science theoretical frameworks that help explain current (and predict future) policy and practice. The following three frameworks are especially relevant in providing insights into what factors need to be considered in a food fortification setting:

1 Multiple streams framework

In his investigation of major policy issues undertaken by the US federal government, Kingdon analysed how issues come to be issues, how they come to the attention of policy-makers, how agendas are set, and why ideas 'have their time' (53). Kingdon conceptualized policy-making as involving three major policy 'streams'. The three streams are:

i) problem stream, consisting of information about real world problems that is derived from data, events, or feedback from past interventions

ii) policy stream, consisting of a policy community of researchers, advocates and other specialists, who analyse problems and formulate possible solutions and alternatives that must be technically feasible and compatible with dominant values

iii) political stream, that sets the governmental agenda and consists of such factors as public opinion, elections, and leadership contests.

Kingdon's theoretical approach is that these three major policy streams tend to be omnipresent during the day-to-day operations of the government and operate independently of each other. At critical times the three streams converge, i.e. a problem is identified and evidence is collected and brought to the government's attention, solutions are proposed (actors and activities, e.g. framing) and the political climate is receptive, and a window of opportunity is opened during which time major policy changes can occur (agendas setting the scene). Conversely, a strong evidence base, represented by the problem stream, in isolation, is unlikely to stimulate the policy-making process. Policy entrepreneurs are at times able to couple these independent streams and facilitate major policy change (54). For instance, those policy entrepreneurs that have a plan of action and strategies for advancing this plan are well-placed to take advantage of policy windows that result from political lobbying.

2 Advocacy coalition framework

The advocacy coalition framework (ACF) builds on the basic concept of sub-systems by explaining policy change as the product of competition between several 'advocacy coalitions' (55). An advocacy coalition is formed with the coming together of individuals and/or groups who share a common belief system that relates to certain policy issues. Scientific evidence is perceived to influence policy through the beliefs of advocacy coalitions who are able to sponsor research, and accept or reject data based on how it aligns with their core beliefs. Policy change is explained as an outcome of fluctuations in the dominant belief systems within a given policy subsystem over time, often many years, and therefore requires sustained advocacy work. These fluctuations are a function of three sets of processes:

i)   The interaction of competing advocacy coalitions within a policy subsystem.

ii) Changes external to the subsystem, such as changes in socioeconomic conditions, changes in governance, and decisions from other policy subsystems.

iii) The effects of 'stable system parameters', such as basic social structure and constitutional rules on the constraints and resources of various actors.

Although accepting the theoretical rigour of the ACF, some policy scientists are proposing additional dimensions and factors to extend its relevance to contemporary settings and dynamics. For example, Shanahan et al. (56), using the ACF as a 'ground spring' for a narrative policy framework, have added narrative analysis as a causal determinant of policy change. The critical contribution of this narrative policy framework is that it proposes that policy narratives are strategically constructed to influence policy change and outcomes and highlights the need for the policy analysis to be especially cognisant of the framing of policy problems and solutions.

3 Network approach

The Network approach to explaining policy-making takes as its starting point the understanding that: 'The model of a unitary, state-centered hierarchical political decision-making structure has always been a fiction, quite remote from real-life decision-making' (57). There are many different understandings of network governance approaches. For this investigation, it is a set of tools used to analyse policy dynamics in a context characterized by a shift from policy being made by a sole actor (centralized government) to policy made through governance arrangements. In this policy context, government is seen as one of many actors.

The network approach emphasizes the interdependent relationships between actors across public and private sectors. Key to analysis is understanding who are the actors involved and what are their relationships and activities. The network approach attempts to explain how actors behave within networks and how factors within and external to networks are connected in determining policy-making (57).

In their ideal form, networks are seen as facilitating exchange of information and sharing of resources in a non-hierarchical fashion. They are understood to be a stabilizing network of linkages, bringing together private and public sectors in relationships that avoid dominance of either sector. In practice, challenges to these partnerships include lack of transparency and uneven distributions of power and accountability. The complex policy environment offers opportunity for some actors to dominate the shape of policy through networks.

Insights from theoretical frameworks to inform policy analysis

If we are to strengthen food fortification policy and practice into the future, we need to understand and learn how, and why, it currently is being made. The policy-making theories and models briefly reviewed in this section reveal that theoretical understandings of policy-making have become progressively more sophisticated. Initially, the policy sciences operated to an optimistic, albeit idealistic, conceptualization of policy-making as a rational-linear process. Then there was clear recognition that irrespective of the quantity and quality of evidence available, it does not speak for itself. The mitigating influences of political and social factors on the translation of evidence into policy were incorporated into various research utilization theories. Finally, the political nature of the policy-making process is reflected in the playing out of the competing rationalities towards public health among actors. Scientific evidence (and ethics) is perceived as not just informing policy decisions, but also can at times be an integral component of the process to privilege and/or diminish the arguments of different stakeholders.

Emerging from this brief review of relevant theories and models of evidence-informed public health policy-making are several insights which informed the critical policy analysis of the case studies in ways that helped explain how and why food fortification policy was made. Although these theoretical frameworks are distinct in the dynamics and mechanisms they provide to explain the policy-making process, they share several common features. They are all based on the premise that the use of evidence is value-laden and that the policy-making process is inherently political. Also, they commonly highlight three variables that are necessary to explain policy-making phenomena. Independently and in combination, these three variables act to influence the way that evidential and ethical evaluative frameworks are interpreted and applied to protect and promote public health and safety in the food fortification policy process. In the present context, these three explanatory variables are:

1 Actors: actors are those individuals or organizations who act in and on the structures and processes involved with food fortification policy-making.

2 Activities: activities are the actions undertaken by actors when acting in and on the structures and processes involved with food fortification policy-making.

3 Agendas: agendas are the underpinning developments and forces shaping the food regulation environment within which food fortification policy is made.

Conclusion

In the complex and vexed world of food fortification policy and practice, evaluative frameworks for evidence and ethics can provide a basis for informed and reasoned decision-making. Much investment has been directed towards establishing standardized rules and procedures for evidence-informed guideline development and risk analysis. Evidential frameworks enable the otherwise abstract objective of protecting public health and safety to be applied transparently when planning food fortification interventions. Regarding ethics, in the absence of explicit evaluative frameworks in UN and national decision-making, there are core theoretical principles that can be drawn upon to inform a justificatory approach to ethical considerations in public health policy-making.

Few researchers, policy-makers, or practitioners would dispute that, in principle, evidential and ethical evaluative frameworks are a sensible ideal to pursue for informing food fortification policy-making. These frameworks have an intuitive appeal because they promise rationality and objectivity for the policy-making process. However, the critiques that accompanied the description of the evaluative frameworks in this chapter reveal that they are not immutable. They can operate within different approaches and this will affect what evidence is valued in the construction of the evidence base, as well as the ethical justification they provide to inform policy decisions. Inevitably, evidence and ethics are value-laden and their use in food fortification activities is inherently political. The selected exemplars of contemporary evidence evaluative frameworks as standardized by UN agencies (and many national food authorities) represent particular approaches, and the implications of these and alternative approaches was assessed and analysed for each of the case studies in Chapters 5–7.

This chapter's description of the evidential and ethical evaluative frameworks and the insights that were identified from the review of theories and models of evidence-informed policy-making provided the foundation for the investigative component of the research presented in this book. This information was used to guide the assessment and analysis of each of the case studies and helped to provide answers to this investigation's research questions. The assessment component of each case study was based on the evidence available for public health benefits and risks, as well as ethical considerations associated with all potential policy interventions. The way that evidence evaluative frameworks and ethical justifications were used in the policy-making process for each case study was then analysed to help explain how and why policies were made. Observed differences between the 'ideal' and the reality were analysed and interpreted against theories to help build understandings of food fortification policy-making processes. The research method that structured this investigation is outlined in Chapter 4, but before detailing this method, the actors, actions, and agendas that influence how the evidential and ethical evaluative frameworks are applied in practice are described in the next chapter.

References

1. Oxman A, Lavis J, Fretheim A, Lewin S. SUPPORT tools for evidence-informed health Policymaking (STP) 16: using research evidence in balancing the pros and cons of policies. *Health Research Policy and Systems* 2009; 7 Suppl 1:S16.

2. Arens, U. Spokeswoman for the British Dietetic Association, as quoted in The Independent, Friday 3 February 2012, page 36, Meg Carter, with permission from The Independent, www.independent.co.uk.

3. Lawrence M. Do food regulatory systems protect public health? *Public Health Nutrition* 2009; 12(11):2247–9.

4. Bowen S, Zwi A. Pathways to 'evidence-informed' policy and practice: a framework for action. *PLoS Medicine* 2005; 2(7):e166.

5. Sackett DL, Rosenberg WM, Gray JA, Haynes RB, Richardson WS. Evidence based medicine: what it is and what it isn't. *British Medical Journal* 1996; 312(7023):71–2.

6. Cochrane A. *Effectiveness and efficiency: random reflections on health services.* London: The Nuffield Provincial Hospitals Trust; 1972.

7. Schulz K, Altman D, Moher D. CONSORT 2010 statement: updated guidelines for reporting parallel group randomised trials. *British Medical Journal* 2010; 340:c332.

8. Cook T, Campbell D. *Quasi-experimentation: design and analysis issues for field settings.* Boston, MA: Houghton Mifflin; 1979.

9. Lawrence M, Worsley A. Concepts and guiding principles. In: Lawrence M, Worsley A (eds). *Public health nutrition: from principles to practice.* Sydney and London: Allen and Unwin and Open University Press; 2007, pp. 5–27.

10. Chung M, Balk E, Ip S, Raman G, Yu W, Trikalinos T, *et al.* Reporting of systematic reviews of micronutrients and health: a critical appraisal. *American Journal of Clinical Nutrition* 2009; 89(4):1099–113.

11. Heaney R. Nutrients, endpoints, and the problem of proof. *Journal of Nutrition* 2008; 138(9):1591–5.

12. Blumberg J, Heaney R, Huncharek M, Scholl T, Stampfer M, Vieth R, *et al.* Evidence-based criteria in the nutritional context. *Nutrition Reviews* 2010; 68(8):478–84.

13. Jacobs DJ, Gross M, Tapsell L. Food synergy: an operational concept for understanding nutrition. *American Journal of Clinical Nutrition* 2009; 89(5):1543S–8S.

14. Hambidge K. Micronutrient Bioavailability: Dietary Reference Intakes and a future perspective. *American Journal of Clinical Nutrition* 2010; 91(5):1430S–2S.

15. Fundación Dieta Mediterránea. *Dieta Mediterránea Candidatura a Patrimonio Inmaterial de la Humanidad.* 2010 [cited 10 February 2012]. Available from: http://candidaturadietamediterranea.org/?lang=en.

16. Bach-Faig A, Berry E, Lairon D, Reguant J, Trichopoulou A, Dernini S, *et al.* Mediterranean diet pyramid today. Science and cultural updates. *Public Health Nutrition* 2011; 14(12A):2274–84.

17. World Health Organization Guidelines Review Committee. *WHO handbook for guideline development. Draft March 2010.* Geneva: WHO; 2010 [cited 3 February 2012]. Available from: http://www.who.int/hiv/topics/mtct/grc_handbook_mar2010_1.pdf.

18. Pena-Rosas J, De-Regil L, Rogers L, Bopardikar A, Panisset U. Translating research into action: WHO evidence-informed guidelines for safe and effective micronutrient interventions. *Journal of Nutrition* 2012; 142(1):197S–204S.

19. Higgins J, Green S, (eds). *Cochrane handbook for systematic reviews of interventions. Version 5.0.2.* The Cochrane Collaboration 2009 [cited 21 July 2011]. Available from: www.cochrane-handbook.org.

20. Cochrane Collaboration. Cochrane Collaboration awarded seat on World Health Assembly. 2011 [cited 2 December 2011]. Available from: http://www.cochrane.org/features/cochrane-collaboration-awarded-seat-world-health-assembly.

21. Balshem H, Helfand M, Schunemann H, Oxman A, Kunz R, Brozek J, *et al.* GRADE guidelines: 3. Rating the quality of evidence. *Journal of Clinical Epidemiology* 2011; 64(4):401–6.

22. Petticrew M, Roberts H. Evidence, hierarchies, and typologies: horses for courses. *Journal of Epidemiology and Community Health* 2003; 57(7):527–9.

23. Kraemer K, de Pee S, Badham J. Evidence in multiple micronutrient nutrition: from history to science to effective programs. *Journal of Nutrition* 2012; 142(1):138S–42S.

24. Kumanyika S, Economos C. Prevention of obesity. Finding the best evidence. *World Nutrition Journal of the World Public Health Nutrition Association* 2011; 2(6).

25. Victora CG, Habicht JP, Bryce J. Evidence-based public health: moving beyond randomized trials. *American Journal of Public Health* 2004; 94(3):400–5.

26. Habicht J, Pelto G. Multiple micronutrient interventions are efficacious, but research on adequacy, plausibility, and implementation needs attention. *Journal of Nutrition* 2012; 142(1):205S–9S.

27. World Health Organization/Food and Agriculture Organization. *Application of risk analysis to food standards issues.* Report of the Joint FAO/WHO Expert Consultation. Geneva; 1995.

28. Codex Alimentarius Commission. *Joint FAO/WHO food standards programme, Codex Alimentarius Commission, procedural manual.* Rome; 2010 [cited 16 December 2011]. Available from: ftp://ftp.fao.org/codex/Publications/ProcManuals/Manual_19e.pdf.

29. Baines J, Cunningham J, Leemhuis C, Hambridge T, Mackerras D. Risk assessment to underpin food regulatory decisions: an example of public health nutritional epidemiology. *Nutrients* 2011; 3(1):164–85.

30. Codex Alimentarius Commission. *REP 11/NFSDU: report of the thirty third session of the Codex committee on nutrition and foods for special dietary uses*. World Health Organization: Geneva; 2010.

31. Codex Alimentarius Commission. *Codex Alimentarius Commission, Procedural Manual*. World Health Organization: Geneva; 2011.

32. Allen L, de Benoist B, Dary O, Hurrell R. *Guidelines on food fortification with micronutrients*. Geneva: World Health Organization; 2006 [cited 25 September 2012]. Available from: http://www.who.int/nutrition/publications/guide_food_fortification_micronutrients.pdf.

33. FOOD STANDARDS AGENCY (2005) The Food Standards Agency's approach to regulatory decision-making: Policy statement for consultation (p.3), Food Standards Agency http://www.food.gov.uk/multimedia/pdfs/approachdecision.pdf Accessed: 28 October 2012.

34. Flynn A, Moreiras O, Stehle P, Fletcher R, Muller D, Rolland V. Vitamins and minerals: a model for safe addition to foods. *European Journal of Nutrition* 2003; 42(2):118–30.

35. Meltzer H, Aro A, Andersen N, Koch B, Alexander J. Risk analysis applied to food fortification. *Public Health Nutrition* 2003; 6(3):281–91.

36. Holland S. *Public health ethics*. Cambridge: Polity Press; 2007.

37. Carter S, Rychetnik L, Lloyd B, Kerridge I, Baur L, Bauman A, *et al*. Evidence, ethics, and values: a framework for health promotion. *American Journal of Public Health* 2011; 101(3):465–72.

38. Childress J, Faden R, Gaare R, Gostin L, Kahn J, Bonnie R, *et al*. Public health ethics: mapping the terrain. *Journal of Law, Medicine and Ethics* 2002; 30(2):170–8.

39. Turoldo F. Responsibility as an ethical framework for public health interventions. *American Journal of Public Health* 2009; 99(7):1197–202.

40. Breton E, De Leeuw E. Theories of the policy process in health promotion research: a review. *Health Promotion International* 2011; 26(1):82–90.

41. Maxwell J. *Qualitative research design: an interactive approach*. California, CA: Sage Publications Inc; 2005.

42. Lasswell H. *The decision process*. College Park, MD: University of Maryland Press; 1956.

43. Weiss C. The many meanings of research utilization. *Public Administration Review* 1979; 5:426–31

44. Hanney S, Gonzalez-Block M, Buxton M, Kogan M. The utilisation of health research in policy-making: concepts, examples and methods of assessment. *Health Research Policy and Systems* 2003; 1(1):2.

45. Choi B. Understanding the basic principles of knowledge translation. *Journal of Epidemiology and Community Health* 2005; 59(2):93.

46. Davies H, Nutley S, Walter I. Why 'knowledge transfer' is misconceived for applied social research. *Journal of Health Services Research and Policy* 2008; 13(3):188–90.

47. Lomas J. Using 'linkage and exchange' to move research into policy at a Canadian foundation. *Health Affairs (Millwood)* 2000; 19(3):236–40.

48. Brownson R, Royer C, Ewing R, McBride T. Researchers and policymakers; travelers in parallel universes. *American Journal of Preventive Medicine* 2006; 30(2):164–72.

49. Innvaer S, Gunn V, Trommald M, Oxman A. Health policy-makers' perceptions of their use of evidence: a systematic review. *Journal of Health Services Research and Policy* 2002; 7:239–44.

50. Campbell DM, Redman S, Jorm L, Cooke M, Zwi AB, Rychetnik L. Increasing the use of evidence in health policy: practice and views of policy makers and researchers. *Australia and New Zealand Health Policy* 2009; 6:21.

51. SUPPORT website. Available from: http://www.support-collaboration.org.

52. Sabatier P. The need for better theories. In: Sabatier P (ed). *Theories of the policy process*, 2 ed. Boulder, CO: Westview; 2007, pp. 3–17.

53. Kingdon J. *Agendas, alternatives and public policies*, 2nd ed. New York: HarperCollins College; 2005.

54. Rütten A, Gelius P, Abu-Omar K. Policy development and implementation in health promotion—from theory to practice: the ADEPT model. *Health Promotion International* 2011; 26(3).

55. Sabatier P, Jenkins-Smith H. *Policy change and learning: an advocacy coalition approach*. Boulder, CO: Westview Press; 1993.

56. Shanahan E, Jones M, McBeth M. Policy narratives and policy processes. *Policy Studies Journal* 2011; 39(3):535–61.

57. Adam S, Kriesi H. The network approach. In: Sabatier P (ed). *Theories of the policy process*. 2 ed. Boulder, CO: Westview; 2007, pp. 129–54.

Chapter 3

Food fortification politics: the actors, activities, and agendas

In an ideal world, health policy would be formulated in a rational, linear process, moving from data collection . . . to scientific consensus . . . Translating science to policy is far messier and convoluted, involving as it does societal priorities, resource allocation, opportunity costs, changing cultural mores, special interests, politics, prejudice, and pure greed (1).

Reproduced with permission from Alfred Sommer, How Public Health Policy Is Created: Scientific Process and Political Reality, American Journal of Epidemiology, 154, (12), p. S4, Oxford University Press, Copyright ©2001 by the Johns Hopkins University Bloomberg School of Public Health.

Introduction

Food is political. Leading food policy analysts have consistently demonstrated that the structure and operation of the food system, from food production to food marketing and purchasing, is influenced by battles among actors with competing values, beliefs, and interests (2, 3). Food fortification is an especially contested topic within the food system because policy-makers must contend with conceptual, vested interest, and technical challenges. Conceptual challenges arise when there may be different views among actors about the cause of a policy problem and whether food fortification or an alternative policy option is the preferred solution. Vested interest challenges arise when various actors have different motivations for supporting or opposing food fortification activities. There may be different motivations between actors with either public health or commercial interests for undertaking food fortification. Food fortification can be a powerful technology for protecting public health and an attractive intervention for food marketers, especially when voluntarily fortified foods can be promoted with appealing nutrient claims. Balancing these often conflicting interests has an added challenge for policy-makers, in that they are reliant on the private sector to prepare and distribute fortified foods. Technical challenges arise when there are practicalities to take into account with applying food fortification policy recommendations to the food supply, e.g. determining which foods can and cannot be fortified, at what levels, with what nutrients, and with what marketing claims.

Food fortification policy-making occurs within food regulatory systems. In the previous chapter, the evidential and ethical evaluative frameworks that inform food fortification decisions within these systems were described. Despite the investment in developing such frameworks, of themselves they cannot drive food fortification policy. Nor can they account for the political dimension that helps explain how and why food fortification activities take place. The review of prominent policy science theoretical frameworks in the previous chapter provided insights to help explain this political dimension and guide the investigation's research design. In practical terms, the theoretical insights emphasize that the food fortification policy-making process cannot be isolated from the myriad actors (i.e. organizations, groups, and individuals who act in the policy processes), activities and agendas operating within and upon food regulatory systems. Therefore, an understanding of food fortification policy and programmes requires a basic appreciation of who these actors are, what activities they undertake and how agendas influence the structure and operation of food regulatory systems. As Walt comments: '... since processes do not have a life of their own, but are dependent on actors to give them expression, analysis of the policy process is interwoven with an exploration of which actors are involved, and how far each may be exerting influence on policy' (4).

This chapter provides a description of the principal actors, activities, and agendas that are involved with food fortification politics. After presenting an overview of the political nature of food fortification in its first section, the chapter is then organized around a brief outline of the food regulatory systems within which food fortification activities are planned, implemented, and (sometimes) evaluated. The chapter's second section focuses on national food regulatory systems. It is not feasible to cover the details of all national food regulatory systems and their peculiar features in this chapter. Instead, a description of the principal actors, activities, and agendas of a generic national food regulatory system is provided. Then the third section of the chapter describes the global food regulatory system's principal actors, activities, and agendas.

The political nature of food fortification
Competing views towards food fortification

Fortified foods are not only potentially powerful products for public health policy interventions but also comprise a substantial and increasing share in the estimated US$ four trillion global food retail sales (5). Food fortification spans many political agendas and attracts many actors. There are contested values, beliefs, and interests among stakeholders about whether food fortification should or should not happen, in what form, and with what technical provisions. These contested views can take a diversity of forms. Some stakeholders might value protecting the so-called 'nutrient integrity', i.e. the 'natural' nutrient composition, of foods, other stakeholders might value innovation and seek out the opportunity to manipulate the nutrient composition of foods. Some stakeholders might believe that food fortification offers the best solution to a policy problem, other stakeholders might believe that an alternative policy intervention would be preferable. Some stakeholders might have a commercial interest in seeking regulatory provisions that permit greater flexibility for voluntary food fortification of their food products, other stakeholders might have a public health interest in seeking regulatory provisions that tighten up provisions permitting voluntary food fortification policy.

Power relations among food fortification actors

Inevitably there are competitions among actors to have their values, beliefs, and interests prevail in food fortification policy and practice. The resolution of these competitions rarely takes place on a level playing field. There are differential power relations among actors and this affects their opportunities to engage with policy-makers. Power differentials arise particularly from the different amount of resources (time and financial) available to various actors. The amount of available resources influences an actor's capacity to participate in a food fortification policy process and to access policy-makers. It is not uncommon for public health nutritionists and public interest non-government organizations (PINGOs) to struggle to engage with a food regulation policy process. For instance, when an opportunity is presented to participate in a public meeting or to make a submission to a policy process, often they must do so without financial support and juggle the time available to undertake the activity with their 'real' (paid) work. Conversely, for many food manufactures, engagement with food regulation policy processes is core business. It is not unusual, and indeed good business sense, for larger food manufacturers to employ legal advisers and nutritionists with food regulation competencies to assiduously represent the manufacturer's interests in the policy process.

The power differential between public and private sector interests groups when engaging with the international level of food fortification policy-making can be especially stark. For instance, Liese reports that of the 156 transnational actors who have observer status in the Codex Alimentarius Commission (Codex, effectively the international food regulator, see later in this chapter) activities, 70% are private sector interest groups (6).

Inevitably, food fortification is about politics in the sense of the word when was defined by Laswell as: 'Who gets what, when, how' (7).

National food regulatory systems

All fortified foods sold within a country, whether produced domestically or imported, must comply with national food law. National food law comprises legislation that establishes the legal framework for, among other activities, regulating food fortification. Usually the legislation takes the form of an act for creating a national food regulatory system within which food fortification regulation is made. In rare instances, food fortification regulation may come into law via the establishment of a dedicated piece of legislation in the form of a food fortification act or decree. Both models of legislation are accompanied by subordinate regulations which are comprised of two components: policy to provide the overarching direction and intent of food standards, and the food standards themselves that prescribe the technical details relating to the composition and labelling of fortified foods permitted under either legislation model (8). This investigation focuses on the model in which national food law is enacted through the establishment of an overarching food regulatory system rather than the more specific food fortification legislation model.

A national food regulatory system consists of a number of actors, activities, and agendas involved with regulating food fortification. These are discussed separately in the following three subsections.

Actors

Actors involved in national food fortification policy primarily include government departments, statutory agencies, expert or representative committees, and non-government actors with interests that are especially affected by the food fortification policy and programme outcomes. Non-government examples are: food manufacturers (and their representative bodies such as the Grocery Manufacturer's Association in the US), food scientists and technologists, public health and consumer organizations and practitioners, and individual citizens. The national government departments most directly engaged with the food regulatory system are those who have responsibilities that affect the structure and operation of the food system, namely the departments of: health, agriculture, industry, consumer affairs, and trade (or their equivalents). A statutory agency such as Food Standards Australia New Zealand (FSANZ) may be established by a government to serve as an independent expert agency with deferred powers to manage food legislative responsibilities. A government department or statutory agency may not necessarily have in-house expertise to assess food fortification topics. Depending on the topic, there may also be a requirement for consultation and input from external stakeholders. Therefore a government or its statutory agency may establish a food fortification expert and/or representative committee comprising individuals from academic, industry, consumer, and non-government organization (NGO) backgrounds to provide advice or other roles depending on the committee's terms of reference. An expert committee consists of individuals with expertise on matters being considered by the committee. A representative committee consists of individuals who represent one of more actors with an interest in the work being undertaken by the committee.

Food regulation is a powerful policy tool for shaping the structure and operation of components of the food system. Consequently, the agendas of the food regulatory systems are diverse and range from protecting public health to promoting consumer, agriculture, and food industry interests. The profile afforded to different food fortification agendas will vary depending on the positioning of the food regulatory system within the government portfolio. A food regulatory system located within a health department and that falls under the responsibility of a minister for health will likely place highest priority on attending to the health considerations of food fortification regulation. Conversely, a food regulatory system located within an agriculture or industry department may place greater emphasis on accommodating food industry interests, such as greater flexibility towards voluntary food fortification permissions. This emphasis might be reflected in how the protection of public health is interpreted and actioned when regulating food fortification.

Activities

The primary food regulatory system activities are threefold: managing policy principles, setting and varying technical food regulations such as food standards, and overseeing enforcement of the regulations (see Figure 3.1 later in the chapter). In the case of food fortification, the management of policy principles involves establishing principles, such as whether food fortification is permitted, under what circumstances, and with what conditions. These policy principles are then put into practice through their translation into the setting of a new, or variation to an existing, food standard that specifies the technical details with which the manufacturers of fortified foods must comply. Enforcement is about ensuring that the food fortification food standard(s) is implemented as legally required in the marketplace and acting to correct transgressions if and when they arise. Without a well-resourced and capable enforcement activity in place, the integrity of the food regulatory system is undermined.

The governance arrangements for a food regulatory system vary among countries. In some countries, the development of food fortification policy principles, the setting of a food fortification standard, and the enforcement of that food standard are undertaken by the one actor or agency, e.g. the US Food and Drug Administration (FDA). In other countries, these activities may be allocated to different agencies within the food regulatory system, e.g. in Australia and New Zealand there is a separation of policy- and food standards-setting activities between a ministerial council and FSANZ, respectively.

Omnipresent during the operation of the food regulatory system are those actors listed earlier with particular views towards the system's processes and outcomes. Although these actors may operate externally to the official food regulatory system governance arrangements, they can exert significant influence through their advocacy activities and inputs during consultation processes.

Advocacy

Actors undertake a variety of activities to promote their values, beliefs, and interests in policy debates. In the context of this investigation advocacy is an activity designed to gain political commitment, social acceptance, and systems support for a potential policy solution to a policy problem. Depending on their available resources and competencies, actors might undertake a variety of advocacy activities including: commissioning research and using the obtained evidence to support their advocacy campaign, meeting with policy-makers, and using the media and public events to raise awareness of their agenda.

Framing

Framing refers to the application of a group of strategies designed to set and then drive a policy agenda along a path, starting out with giving meaning to a policy problem and how it is represented. Subsequently, framing plays a significant role in influencing how the problem is interpreted, including: its causes, the actors who will best be able to be engaged, and what policies and policy interventions are most appropriate to solve the problem (9). Given the inherently political nature of policy-making, there is a need to be critically aware of the way that a policy problem might be represented to privilege the values, beliefs, and interests of certain actors and obscure those of other actors. The manner in which problems are represented largely predetermines who has power over policy processes, because it plays a role in influencing whose views are perceived as legitimate and heard. Therefore, the ability to use framing to shape how a problem is represented becomes a critical first step in influencing the choice of a preferred policy solution to a policy problem.

Agendas

Food regulatory systems operate as one component of the broad platform of government roles and responsibilities. The structure and operation of a food regulatory system will be shaped by agendas that originate directly from within government, or indirectly from external factors that influence government operations overall. Two particular agendas that shape the operation of national food regulatory systems, one located within government and one located externally, are now described.

Dominant political ideology

In recent decades, the ideology of neoliberalism has come to dominate the policy and regulatory activities of governments in many high-income countries. At its core, neoliberalism is characterized by the idea that a relatively 'small' government presence, the so-called 'light touch' of government, and a relatively large engagement with the marketplace, is an effective and efficient way to govern society. This idea has been acted upon by pursuing a deregulation agenda to promote free trade and reduce perceived impediments to the operations of the private sector. Deregulation is viewed as helping promote greater flexibility for the private sector to innovate in product research and development in order to promote competition and provide increased choice to citizens. It is believed that all else being equal, it is more efficient to manage non-acute public health risks within society through the provision of more consumer information and less regulation. It is not uncommon for actors aligned with this ideological perspective to label regulation with pejorative terms such as 'red tape', implying that it can unnecessarily tie up the activities of the free market. Some actors also assert that the excessive use of regulation risks creating a 'nanny' state in which the government over-protects its citizens.

One example of how this ideology is expressed in a food regulation setting is provided by the UK FSA when it states that, whereas it has a:

> ... statutory objective to protect public health and consumers' other interests in relation to food and drink, it is aware that excessive or unclear regulations can place a burden on business, the public sector and civil society groups ... and so hinder effective delivery of the intended benefits (10).

The agency's website proceeds to state that: there is a 'Reducing regulation programme' which is about: 'making regulations easier for business, the public sector and civil society groups to understand and comply with without compromising public health' (10).

A second example that illustrates how this ideology shapes the approach taken to develop food regulation is the work undertaken by the Australian Department of Finance and Deregulation's Office of Best Practice Regulation (OBPR). The OBPR has a mandate to support an overarching government approach to reducing the regulatory burden on business. The OBPR reviews all the Australian government's policies and regulations for their impact on business via the regulatory impact statement (RIS) process. According to requirements set out in the OBPR's handbook:

> A RIS is mandatory for all decisions made by the Australian government and its agencies that are likely to have a regulatory impact on business or the not-for-profit sector, unless that impact is of a minor or machinery nature and does not substantially alter existing arrangements (11).

What this means in practice is that if the Australian food regulatory system wishes to vary or set food fortification regulation, either mandate food fortification or permit voluntary food fortification, it will be required to prepare a RIS and submit it to the assessment process conducted by OBPR. The food regulatory system must demonstrate that the monetary benefits of the proposed intervention outweigh the costs to business, potentially shaping whether the regulation proceeds or the way that it is constructed. Equivalent assessment requirements for the potential beneficial health, social, and environmental impacts from a proposed food fortification regulation are often overlooked as the regulatory system is required to present such potential impacts as quantifiable causal links even though such relationships are better specified and measured using qualitative approaches.

The extensive nature and scope of the food system means that food policy considerations inevitably cut across many government departments' policy agendas. It would be naïve to assume that food fortification policy-making takes place independently of existing policies or necessarily receives priority attention. It is not unusual to observe public policies operating within a hierarchy, with those policies emanating from a finance department for instance generally having a higher status in decision-making relative to those that relate to public health. The influence of the deregulation policy agenda over the contemporary food regulatory system highlights that those government departments responsible for overarching policy frameworks can have a pervasive, albeit indirect, role in shaping the operations of the food regulatory system. The existence of such policy hierarchies can lead to policy 'disjunctions'. For example, while a government's health department might be promoting healthy food selection behaviours to the community, its industry department might simultaneously be subsidizing the manufacture of high-energy, nutrient-poor foods. Also, its finance department might be permitting the manufacturers of such food products to claim related marketing expenses as a legitimate business expense that can be offset against their tax returns. In response, 'all-of-government' or 'joined-up' approaches to food policy have been proposed, so that such disjunctions might be avoided and opportunities for different government departments to coordinate their policy activities might be better identified and acted upon (12).

Global food trade and international obligations

Food trade among countries is a major economic activity. International governance arrangements have been established to manage global food trade and set frameworks for promoting trade liberalization and removing barriers to the flow of foods. Those countries wishing to participate in global food trade are obliged to ensure that their domestic food policies and regulations abide by their international obligations, for example, responsibilities as required by membership of the World Trade Organization (WTO). WTO rules and provisions that relate to food fortification are legally binding on member countries, even if domestic food fortification regulation must be changed.

The WTO was established in 1995 as the international organization to oversee the operation of the rules of trade between member nations. The core role of the WTO is administering the various WTO agreements which provide a framework for the preparation, adoption, and application of technical regulations. The basic WTO principle that guides the implementation of the agreements is 'non-discrimination'. This means that WTO members cannot discriminate, for example, between their partners trading in fortified foods, or between imported and locally-produced fortified foods that are otherwise similar. The main WTO agreements that impact on health policies and programmes are the agreement on sanitary and phytosanitary measures (SPS) and the agreement on technical barriers to trade (TBT). The SPS agreement contains specific rules for countries wanting to restrict trade to ensure food safety and the protection of human life from plant- or animal-carried diseases (the latter are termed zoonoses). The main purpose of the SPS agreement is to restrict the use of technical regulations and conformance procedures as disguised trade barriers (13). Instead, sanitary or phytosanitary requirements need to be necessary and scientifically justifiable. The provisions of the TBT agreement are especially relevant to food fortification considerations. Under the TBT agreement, all WTO members have the right to use technical regulations to restrict trade for legitimate objectives. The protection of human health or safety is one such legitimate objective. However, there are strict conditions that apply if a country proposes to restrict trade on the basis of protecting human health and safety. According to article 2.2 of the TBT agreement, when considering health protection in preparing technical regulations, unnecessary obstacles to international trade must be avoided by ensuring that the regulations are not more 'trade-restrictive than necessary to fulfil a legitimate objective, taking account of the risks non-fulfilment would create' (13).

The obligation to abide by the WTO agreements presents challenges for the planning and implementation of domestic food fortification policies and programmes. What might be considered a reasonable food trade restriction on public health grounds? For example, a country might want to restrict the importation of voluntarily-fortified foods, or conversely require certain imported foods to be fortified with a particular nutrient. These approaches are technical regulations that fall under the TBT agreement. They are powerful regulatory approaches to target the composition and supply of certain foods. However, they may be assessed as being more trade-restrictive than necessary to protect human health or safety, and are vulnerable to accusations of being discriminatory.

There is no 'recipe' as such for a country wishing to develop a food fortification regulatory approach to protect human health and safety, while fully participating in global food trade. Whether or not a regulatory approach to support (or restrict) a food fortification activity is justified will depend upon building a case that fulfils the procedural requirements set down in the relevant WTO agreement (14). The favourable assessment of food fortification regulatory approaches that fall under the TBT agreement is predicated on demonstrating their integral role in contributing to the protection of human health or safety. Moreover, it needs to be demonstrated that the approach(es) are not more trade-restrictive than necessary to protect human health or safety, taking account of the risks non-fulfilment would create. In recognition of the vexed nature of how the protection of human health or safety might be interpreted and applied against food trade objectives within the context of WTO agreements, the World Health Organization (WHO) and WTO in 2002 published a joint study addressing this topic (15). Notably, a narrow approach to what was considered legitimate human health or safety concerns was documented. Whereas the study recognized immediate safety issues as legitimate concerns for food trade, it was more circumspect about the legitimacy of nutrition considerations such as the risk of promoting dietary imbalances resulting from food trade.

A complex pattern of interactions occurs among the principal actors, activities, and agendas for a generic national food regulatory system. A simplified version of this interplay is represented in Figure 3.1.

Global food regulatory system

The food system is increasingly global in scale. The efficient operation of the global food system requires the harmonization of national food laws and regulations, operating procedures, and outcomes as much as possible. The WTO agreements address trade aspects of the global food system and they, along with other international obligations, impact on national food regulatory systems. However, their role is not concerned primarily with health and safety, or quality aspects of food law and regulation, a dedicated global food regulatory system is required. An additional rationale for a global food regulatory system is that many low- to middle-income countries (LMICs) lack the resources and

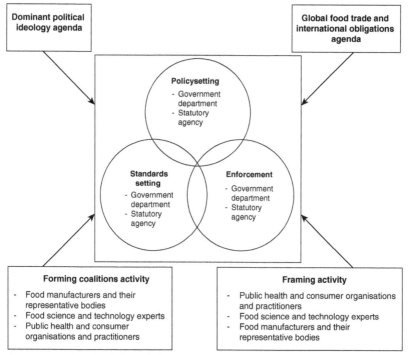

Fig. 3.1 The principal actors, activities, and agendas for a national food regulatory system.

capacity to: fully establish national food regulatory systems, collect scientific evidence, and conduct a scientific assessment process to undertake food regulation policy development, implementation, and evaluation. Instead, they often defer to United Nation (UN) agencies, and in particular Codex, to support them in their food regulation activities (16).

Codex effectively has become the world body responsible for setting food standards. Codex was established by the Food and Agricultural Organization (FAO) and the WHO in 1963 to implement the joint FAO/WHO food standards programme. Codex develops harmonized international food standards, guidelines, and codes of practice, and promotes coordination of all food standards work undertaken by international governmental and NGOs (17). Article 1 of the Codex statutes states that the primary purpose of the of the joint FAO/WHO food standards programme is: 'protecting the health of the consumers and ensuring fair practices in the food trade' (18).

The Codex Alimentarius (meaning food code) is a collection of internationally adopted food standards, guidelines, codes of practice, and other recommendations, that is considered the global reference for national food regulators, food producers and processors, citizens, and decision-makers involved with international food trade (18). Although Codex standards are advisory and not internationally enforceable, regularly they provide the benchmark for national legislation. Indeed, the UN recognized the importance of Codex in addressing food safety internationally in 1985, when it passed resolution 39/248 that advised that when formulating national food policies, governments should support and adopt standards from Codex (19). More recently, the WTO's SPS agreement requires WTO members to base their sanitary and phytosanitary measures on international standards and to participate in Codex. The SPS agreement specifically recognizes Codex texts as the international benchmark. The TBT agreement indirectly references Codex texts. Thus, Codex standards directly affect food safety and the resolution of many trade disputes associated with international food commerce (20).

Risk analysis procedures are central to the formulation of Codex food safety standards (see Chapter 2). Codex reports that it is this scientific basis to its texts that explains why they are regarded as the international reference for food safety standards by the WTO (17). Member countries may adopt standards with a higher level of health protection than those in the Codex Alimentarius; however, such standards must be scientifically based and not used unjustifiably to prevent trade.

Codex is responsible for setting international policy principles for food fortification. The original Codex principles for the addition of essential nutrients to foods were published in 1987 and subsequently amended in 1989 and 1991 (21). As explained in the introduction to this book, Codex recognizes four purposes for adding nutrients to foods: restoration, equivalence, special purpose food composition, and fortification. A risk analysis framework was not included in these Codex principles. At its 31st session the CCNFSDU stated that the purpose of the revision was to extend the Codex principles for adding nutrients to food (22). In effect the revision is preparing Codex principles that will enable food manufacturers to undertake a greater variety and extent of voluntary food fortification. In revising the principles to open up more opportunities for voluntary food fortification, the CCNFSDU is proposing that it can protect public health by putting in place a risk analysis procedure. A consultation on the structure and on the text of the principles in the document being revised was undertaken in the lead up to the CCNFSDU's 34th session (in 2012). Despite the public health importance of this policy development process, Codex observer participation during the consultation period involved only food and/or supplement industries and no public health or consumer organizations (23).

The governance of the global food regulatory system operates on a larger scale and with more actors than that in place for national food regulatory systems. In common with the activities of actors at the national level, actors at the global level also participate in forming coalitions and framing policy topics. The description of these general activities is not repeated here.

In the next section, first the principal UN agencies and then the principal non-UN actors engaged with food fortification and their particular food regulation activities are described. The numerous non-UN actors are organized into six categories: academic/research institutes, bilateral donors, multilateral donors, multisectoral collaborations, NGOs, and private philanthropists. A prominent actor(s) in each of these categories will be profiled to illustrate the contribution of the relevant category to food fortification. Then the primary agenda that is shaping food fortification activities at the global level, global health governance and the pursuit of public–private partnerships, briefly will be discussed in the context of what it means for food fortification.

Actors and their activities

Principal United Nation actors

Food and Agriculture Organization The FAO's mandate is to: 'raise levels of nutrition, improve agricultural productivity, better the lives of rural populations and contribute to the growth of the world economy' (24). The FAO's main activities in international food regulation are exercised through its role in collaborating with the WHO to manage the joint FAO/WHO food standards programme. Its specific food fortification-related roles include coordinating and maintaining: food and nutrition country profiles, the analysis of food composition data, and nutrition assessments and monitoring such as 'State of food insecurity in the world' reports and FAO statistical databases on foods available for consumption.

In its policy statement entitled: 'Fortification of food with micronutrients' (25), the FAO describes its role in providing technical assistance to governments to support food fortification activities. The policy statement provides a perspective that places the effectiveness of food fortification into a context that is rarely explicitly stated by other actors involved in food fortification. It explains that FAO views food fortification programmes by themselves as having certain limitations. These limitations include: that the population groups most in need of improved nutrition are the poor who have low purchasing power for fortified foods, that poor population groups present with multiple micronutrient deficiencies which cannot necessarily be addressed by fortified foods, and that the technology for food fortification requires ongoing development. Based on this perspective, the FAO believes that food fortification programmes need to be implemented as a part of a comprehensive micronutrient malnutrition reduction strategy. Such a strategy should include: 'Poverty reduction programmes along with agricultural, health, education, and social intervention programmes to promote consumption of nutritious foods by all, but in particular by the nutritionally vulnerable'.

United Nations Children's Fund The United Nations Children's Fund (UNICEF) is mandated to advocate for the protection of children's rights, to help meet their basic needs, and to expand their opportunities to reach their full potential. Nutrition, incorporating food fortification activities, is one of the eight key programme areas implied in UNICEF's medium-term strategic framework, and there is a particular focus on the treatment of severe malnutrition (26). UNICEF works with governments in both donor and developing countries to develop food fortification programmes, and has been particularly active in supporting the implementation of universal salt iodization and wheat flour fortification. UNICEF's food fortification work is informed by WHO recommendations and scientific evidence on micronutrient deficiency. This work includes aiding research into micronutrient deficiencies, offering technical support such as implementing pilot projects for local governments, and advocating for the development of food fortification legislation and regulatory frameworks.

World Food Programme The World Food Programme (WFP) coordinates the UN food aid activities by using food to meet emergency needs and to support economic and social development. It describes itself as the: 'World's largest humanitarian agency fighting hunger' (27). Whereas UNICEF focuses on severe malnutrition, WFP has the mandate to address moderate malnutrition and thereby aims to help reduce the incidence of severe malnutrition (27). The WFP has been active in distributing fortified staple foods and condiments as components of its work programme for many years. Recently, it has been working with partners in the private sector, universities, UN, and NGOs to develop and assess the effectiveness of the following five 'special nutritional products', which represent extensions of more conventional fortified foods (27):

1 Fortified blended foods: are mixtures of cereals, soya beans, and pulses fortified with vitamins and minerals. They are designed to provide extra protein and micronutrients in food assistance programmes in addition to the general ration.

2 Ready-to-use foods: are formulated to meet the nutritional needs of young (6–59 months) and moderately malnourished children. They may contain vegetable fat, dry skimmed milk, maltodextrin, sugar, and whey. They are used mostly in emergency situations to supplement breastmilk and other food.

3 High energy biscuits: are high-energy density and fortified with vitamins and minerals. They are ideal for use in the first days of an emergency.

4 Micronutrient powder or 'Sprinkles': is a tasteless powder containing the recommended daily intake of 16 micronutrients for one person. It can be sprinkled onto home-prepared food after cooking just before eating and is useful when the fortification of cereal flour cannot be implemented or when it is inadequate for specific groups.

5 Compressed food bars: are bars of compressed food containing baked wheat flour, vegetable fat, sugars, soya protein concentrate, and malt extract. They are used in disaster relief operations when local food cannot be distributed or prepared. They should not be used for children younger than six months or during the first two weeks of treatment of severe malnutrition.

World Health Organization The WHO directs and coordinates health-related activities within the UN system. The organization describes its responsibilities as: providing leadership on global health matters, shaping health research, setting standards, describing evidence-based policy options, providing technical support to countries, and monitoring and assessing health (28). The WHO's main activities in international food regulation are exercised through its role in collaborating with the FAO to manage the joint FAO/WHO food standards programme.

The Department of Nutrition for Health and Development (NHD) coordinates nutrition activities within WHO, including those that relate to food fortification. The NHD has organized its work programme into four strategic areas: nutrition policy and scientific advice, growth assessment and surveillance, micronutrients, and nutrition in the life course (28). The following objectives and WHO food fortification-related activities are associated with the micronutrients strategic area:

Objectives:

1 To monitor the vitamin and mineral status of populations globally.

2 To help member states and their partners design and implement effective strategies to achieve vitamin and mineral balance in diets.

3 To advocate for the importance of vitamins and minerals in health and nutrition.

Principal WHO food fortification-related activities that support these objectives:

1 Surveillance of micronutrient deficiencies: the vitamin and mineral nutrition information system was established in 1991 following a request by the World Health Assembly (WHA) to strengthen surveillance of micronutrient

deficiencies at the global level. Its micronutrients database compiles national, within-country regional, and first-administrative level data on vitamin and mineral nutritional status of populations in countries. These data are used to generate estimates of the global burden of disease and the contribution of vitamin and mineral deficiencies as risk factors for premature mortality, disability, and loss of health (29).

2   Evidence-informed guidelines: an example of a WHO evidence-informed food fortification guideline is the 2009 'Recommendations on wheat and maize flour fortification meeting report: interim consensus statement' (30).

3   Technical assistance for undertaking food fortification programmes: in 2006, WHO and FAO published the manuscript: 'Guidelines on food fortification with micronutrients' to assist countries to undertake food fortification programmes (7).

4   Online resource library: in August 2011, the WHO launched its electronic library of evidence for nutrition actions (eLENA) (31), designed to serve as a centralized and easily accessible web-based resource for interested actors to link to WHO evidence-informed nutrition guidelines and the underlying evidence for nutrition interventions, including food fortification. It is intended that eLENA will be a resource to support countries to implement and scale-up food fortification (and other nutrition) interventions.

Principal non-United Nation actors

Academic/research institutes Academic/research institutes undertake research to provide knowledge for decision-makers to formulate food fortification activities to protect and promote public health. They form partnerships on food fortification activities at various times with UN agencies. Globally, a leading academic/research institute that contributes to food fortification policy debates is the International Food Policy Research Institute (IFPRI). Among its many activities, IFPRI undertakes research to provide knowledge relevant to policymakers on how to reduce poverty and improve the food security of populations in LMICs, and thereby help end hunger and malnutrition (32). IFPRI jointly coordinates HarvestPlus (33), which is developing and distributing seeds for biofortified crops as a low-cost and sustainable approach to reduce global micronutrient malnutrition. Biofortification involves selecting and breeding staple crop varieties to have a relatively high vitamin and mineral composition and superior agronomic qualities.

Bilateral donors Bilateral donors are national agencies that donate funds directly to LMIC governments, as well as partnering with UN and non-UN agencies in undertaking activities. There are many countries with agencies involved in bilateral donor food fortification programmes. A prominent example of an actor within this category is the US Agency for International Development (USAID). USAID is the official federal agency within the US government by which development assistance is provided to LMICs (34). Its food fortification activities are undertaken utilizing the private sector in micronutrient programmes where feasible. For example, at the 2011 world economic forum in Davos, Switzerland, USAID signed a memorandum of understanding with DSM Nutritional Products, the world's largest manufacturer of micronutrients and vitamins, to support food fortification activities in LMICs starting with rice fortification in countries such as Bangladesh, Cambodia, Ghana, Mali, Senegal, and Tanzania (34).

Multilateral donors Multilateral donors are organizations that combine donors' funds and distribute them for projects in LMICs. There are several large multilateral donors involved in food fortification activities. The example of a prominent actor and its activities in this category is the World Bank. The World Bank is a source of financial and technical assistance to developing countries around the world. It provides low-interest loans, interest-free credits, and grants to developing countries for a wide array of purposes that include investments in food fortification programmes (35). According to the World Bank: 'No other technology [food fortification] offers as large an opportunity to improve lives at such low cost and in such a short time' (36).

Non-government organizations The term NGO broadly refers to non-state, not-for-profit, voluntary organizations that nonetheless usually have a formal structure. There are two main types of NGO: those that represent public sector interests, i.e. PINGOs, and those that represent business sector interests, i.e. business interest non-government organizations (BINGOs). One example of each of these types follows.

The Micronutrient Initiative (MI) is an example of an international PINGO actively promoting food fortification and supplementation interventions. Established in 1992, following the pledge of the 1990 world summit for children to protect children against malnutrition, it functioned initially as a secretariat within the International Development Research Centre (IDRC) in Canada, and now has evolved to be a Canadian-based NGO (37). It describes itself as being: 'The leading organization working exclusively to eliminate vitamin and mineral deficiencies in the world´s most vulnerable populations' (38). MI carries out the following work in partnership with governments, foundations, the private sector, and multilateral agencies: aiding governments, food producers and partner organizations to plan, implement, and evaluate programmes that deliver micronutrients to people who need them most, providing fiscal and technical assistance, including offering procurement and quality control of supplies and equipment, and educating government and advocating about vitamin and mineral programmes.

MI's funding is derived from a range of sources. In its 2010–2011 annual report, it lists its funding sources as: Asian Development Bank, Centers for Disease Control and Prevention (CDC) Foundation, Children's Investment Fund Foundation (UK), China National Salt Industry Corporation, Dow Chemical Company Foundation, DSM Nutritional Products, FHI 360, Global Alliance for Improved Nutrition (GAIN), the government of Canada, through the Canadian International Development agency (CIDA), Helen Keller International, Inter-American Development Bank, Irish Aid, Izumi Foundation, Kiwanis International, Mathile Institute for the Advancement of Human Nutrition, Project Healthy Children, Salt Institute, Teck Resources, UNICEF, US Fund for UNICEF, World Bank, and WFP (38).

Sight and Life is a humanitarian initiative of DSM Nutritional Products and an example of an international BINGO actively promoting food fortification and supplementation interventions. Reference to the word 'sight' in its name relates to its original role in combating vitamin A deficiency in the developing world when it was founded in founded in 1986. It now works to reduce all forms of micronutrient deficiency by collaborating with universities and global and local partners, including the Flour Fortification Initiative (FFI), GAIN, WFP, and WHO (39). DSM Nutritional Products is the world's leading supplier of vitamins, carotenoids, and other chemicals to the feed, food, pharmaceutical, and personal care industries (40).

Private philanthropists There are a number of private philanthropic organizations that provide support for food fortification activities. The Bill and Melinda Gates Foundation is one of the world's largest private philanthropic organizations. Most of its work is done through grants provided to partners in self-defined priority areas. The Foundation reports that in 2009 alone it paid approximately US$ three billion in grants and an additional US$72 million in direct charitable contributions (41). Actors to whom the Foundation provides substantial grants are GAIN in the area of food fortification and HarvestPlus in the area of biofortification. Food fortification is regarded by the foundation as an especially promising intervention to tackle micronutrient deficiencies. Bill Gates, the co-founder of the Foundation, has been quoted as saying: 'Fortifying foods with basic vitamins and minerals is both essential and affordable' (42).

Public–private partnerships Public–private partnerships (PPPs) are described by the WHO as collaborations between public and private sector actors that vary according to participants, legal status, governance, management, policy-setting prerogatives, contributions, and operational roles to achieve specific goals and outcomes (43). PPPs are the primary agenda-influencing global food fortification governance arrangements and are now discussed. Two particularly prominent examples of PPPs involved in global food fortification activities, GAIN and FFI, are described.

The Swiss-based GAIN was launched at the UN general assembly special session on children in May 2002 as a global and regional non-profit alliance of public, private, and civic groups committed to eliminating micronutrient deficiencies. It works with UN agencies and receives funding from a number of public and private sector donors, including the Bill and Melinda Gates Foundation and USAID. In turn, GAIN's Business Alliance (44) supports PPPs involving major global food and beverage companies, including: Coca-Cola, Cargill, Danone, Mars Inc, PepsiCo, Unilever, and Kraft, to stimulate market-based solutions that address global malnutrition. Its objective is to mobilize US$700 million of private-sector investment to fight malnutrition through this business alliance (45).

GAIN is the primary vehicle globally brokering among governments, NGOs, the private sector, and civil society to promote food fortification. Its goal is: 'To reach more than one billion people with fortified foods that have sustainable nutritional impact' (46). Shortly after its launch, the then executive director for GAIN stated: 'Now the challenge before us is how do we fortify food as fast as we can?' (47). At the national level, GAIN provides assistance grants and technical advice to support the delivery of fortified foods. These activities are coordinated by national fortification alliances comprised of the government, food manufacturers, and producers, and consumer groups (48). It reports that since 2002, it has scaled up 36 large collaborations in 25 countries so that 400 million people are now being exposed to fortified food products (46). For example, it has invested in projects that launched fortified: soy sauce in China, fish sauce in Vietnam, cottonseed oil in Côte d'Ivoire, wheat flour in Morocco, and maize flour in South Africa (49).

The FFI is a partnership arrangement involving a network of individuals, private organizations, public entities, academic institutions, and civic groups working together to make flour fortification a standard milling practice worldwide. At the national level, the FFI serves as a catalyst for partnerships which encourage flour fortification. It works by building alliances between governments and international agencies, wheat and flour milling corporations, and consumer and civic organizations. In this regard, it describes itself as a: 'Public-private-civic investment in each nation' (50). FFI works with UN agencies and among the actors already mentioned it receives funding from the Bill and Melinda Gates Foundation and GAIN.

Since 2004, the FFI has helped increase the amount of fortified flour produced by roller mills globally from 18% to 30% (51). It has contributed to this achievement by providing sophisticated resources, such as information for interested people in countries that are not fortifying flour to create a national food fortification alliance to advocate for flour fortification, and a resource library with supporting materials and tool kits for millers and premix manufacturers. Also, it has available spokespeople to speak to the media and a technical support group to provide detailed information on the equipment and procedures needed for flour fortification.

The prominent actors involved in food fortification activities at the global (and national) levels of governance are shown in Figure 3.2. The figure depicts the seven main categories of actors and for each category there is at least one prominent actor identified.

These actors act independently and as parts of a web of partnership combinations. An overarching driver of this involvement of actors and their multiple relationships is the changing nature of the global health governance arrangements. These changing arrangements are described in the next section.

Agendas

Global health governance arrangements

Global food fortification activities are taking place within the context of significant and controversial changes to global health governance arrangements.

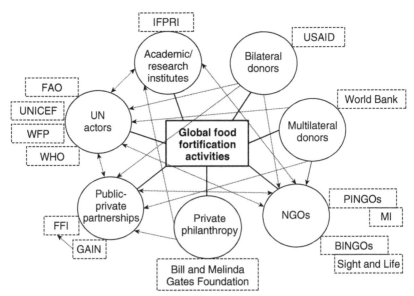

Fig. 3.2 The web of prominent actors and their major partnership interactions involved with global food fortification activities.

Conventionally, it was UN agencies that, for the most part, were responsible for formulating and implementing global food fortification activities. Now it is believed that new and innovative business models and participatory approaches are needed to encourage actors to interact in different ways from the past, so as to be more effective in achieving the Millennium Development Goal (MDG) targets (52). According to the WHO, no single entity has sufficient funding, resources, influence, expertise, or reach to tackle the complex nutrition challenges in communities, at national and regional levels, or worldwide (53). Illustrating this view is the fact that the cost of addressing global malnutrition has been estimated at US$10–12 billion (54), well-beyond the budgetary constraints of the WHO.

Such new governance arrangements are being enacted through a number of mechanisms, including multisectoral collaborations, coalitions, strategic alliances and, in particular, PPPs (described in the previous section) between UN agencies and the private sector and civil society (55). PPPs are having a profound effect on which actors are involved in global health policies and programmes and the activities that they are undertaking. For example, in China UNICEF has partnered with GAIN and the Asian Development Bank to work with the government and private food companies to promote the fortification of staple foods like flour, soy sauce, and salt with iodine, iron, and other nutrients (56). UNICEF has been a strong advocate for PPPs. In its joint publication with MI on the role of PPPs in promoting food fortification, UNICEF states that it is urgent that the world ask food companies to extend their involvement in food fortification as they have the products, technology, distribution channels, and marketing skills to make it happen. (57)

These changes to global health governance arrangements have not occurred overnight. Historically, governments have relied to varying degrees on PPPs and market-driven 'solutions' to address public health nutrition challenges. In recent years, the extent of this approach and its active pursuit within the UN system has dramatically increased (58). In 1993, the WHA called on WHO to explore partnerships with the private sector and NGOs in the implementation of national strategies for health for all (59). Subsequently, WHO's interaction with the commercial sector has broadened and deepened (60). The most well-known partnership is the UN Global Compact. The compact was launched in 1999 by former UN secretary-general Kofi Annan at the world economic forum, with the purpose of stimulating private sector actions to support UN goals. In his 2010 report entitled: 'Keeping the promise: a forward-looking review to promote an agreed action agenda to achieve the MDGs by 2015', presented to the general assembly, UN secretary-general Ban Ki Moon highlighted that the business community had an integral role to play in the achievement of the MDGs by 2015 (61).

Proponents of PPPs present this mechanism for system change as a win–win for the actors involved in food fortification activities (62). For UN agencies, there is the opportunity to access financial resources from the private sector to strengthen their capacity to undertake food fortification activities. In addition, UN agencies may access partners' expertise for product innovation, their communication know-how to raise visibility about pressing issues, and their networks for logistical support and distribution systems. For partners, there are benefits from gaining access to UN services, marketing opportunities for their products, and the goodwill that they receive in being associated with such global food fortification activities.

PPP arrangements are now commonplace in the WHO guideline development process (outlined in Chapter 2). The Micronutrients Unit within the WHO's NHD states that to support the process of formulating evidence-informed food fortification guidelines, it receives grants from the MI, CDC's International Micronutrient Malnutrition Prevention and Control Program (IMMPaCt), GAIN, and the Government of Luxembourg. The unit explains that donors do not: fund specific guidelines, participate in any decision related to the guideline development process, have membership of the guideline groups, or have involvement with the formulation of recommendations (63).

The active pursuit of PPPs in global health governance engenders debate. At the heart of the debate are different views about the respective roles and responsibilities of governments, the private sector, and civil society in protecting and promoting public health. The new governance structures, innovative business models and participatory approaches have created an environment that has raised the influence of PPPs in strategic policy decisions and their implementation. Many people express concern with this development, arguing that the UN agencies and the private sector fundamentally have different objectives and roles. For instance, in their paper published in a special issue of the Standing Committee on Nutrition News dedicated to exploring the vexed topic of how to engage nutrition and business, Brady and Rundall comment:

> The role of governments is to govern in the public interest. The role of executives is to run their corporations within the rules that society places upon them. Given that company executives have a fiduciary duty to maximize shareholder value, government, UN and NGO policy-makers need to be aware that this will sometimes conflict with the public interest, and they must put appropriate safeguards in place (64).

By partnering with the private sector, BINGOs, and PINGOs, the UN agencies and national governments are giving authority to such organizations to be involved in the planning and implementation of public health activities that affect populations. Yet these partners are not subject to the same democratic processes that apply to UN agencies and national governments. One of the core aspects of 'good governance' of any initiative is the representation and participation of those affected by the exercise of power (65). Currently, whether there is an adequate level of this representation and participation for many PPPs is not immediately apparent. This situation raises fundamental questions about the legitimacy of PPPs and their accountability to governments and the citizens affected by their activities.

PPPs place much confidence in the ability of market-driven interventions to solve public health nutrition problems resulting from inadequate dietary nutrient intakes. A core rationale for partnering with the private sector is to enable UN agencies to draw on this sector's product innovations, skills, and delivery networks to supply and distribute fortified foods to help address such problems. Yet in pursuing such partnerships, it is important that there is not an over-reliance on such technological interventions to the oversight of alternative policy interventions. Inadequate dietary nutrient intakes result from a variety of health, social, economic, and environmental causes that require alternative policy interventions, such as agriculture development programmes, poverty alleviation, or social marketing to effectively address the underlying cause of the inadequate dietary nutrient intake. The health impacts of those PPPs that are advocating for food fortification, such as GAIN's business alliance, are yet to be comprehensively and independently evaluated, so it is difficult to understand the benefits and challenges of using a PPP approach to address micronutrient malnutrition. In one of the few available independent evaluations of PPPs more broadly, Buse and Harmer argue that there are a number of concerns with the way that some PPPs currently are operating. The concerns they raise include that PPPs can: skew national priorities of recipient countries by imposing those of donor partners, deprive specific stakeholders a voice in decision-making, and fail to compare the costs and benefits of public versus private interventions (65).

PPPs assume a role in the exercise of power and the challenge for public health interests is that in striving for effective food fortification activities public health objectives are not subverted by commercial objectives (66). Certainly, successful food fortification activities require the cooperation of food manufacturers, and their interests need to be considered in food fortification activities. However, in the context of putting safeguards in place for PPPs, the following excerpt from a UNICEF and MI report about the need for governments to provide incentives to the global grain council in return for its support for food fortification raises the question: 'Are certain actors striking a correct balance in representing public health and commercial interests?:

> The job of government is to create the conditions that make it commercially viable for food companies to take up the challenge of VM [vitamin and mineral] deficiency. For example, governments can:
> - Help build public demand for fortified foods through health and education services, and the print and broadcast media.
> - Assist with start-up finance, technical training, product development, consumer testing, and marketing costs.
> - Endorse approved food products, with official government seals or stamps for use in commercial advertising.
> - Allow distribution of certain fortified foods via schools, hospitals, clinics.
> - Specify fortified foods when placing food orders for schools, the armed forces, health service personnel, or for disaster relief and refugee feeding programmes.
> - These are the kind of public-private partnership deals can make it viable for food companies to invest in developing and marketing fortified products that will be available to the poor (57).

Moreover, shortly before the public launching of GAIN, *The Wall Street Journal* reported that in exchange for their fortified food contributions, GAIN was proposing to assist food companies to lobby for supportive tariffs and tax rates as well as rapid regulatory consideration for new fortified foods in certain countries. It also reported that GAIN would provide funding to local governments to implement marketing campaigns to stimulate demand for fortified foods (67).

Debates about the appropriateness of PPPs often hinge on whether a pragmatic or principled view is taken. Pragmatically, PPPs might be viewed as a necessary approach so as to enable UN agencies to work with those organizations that directly influence what people eat, even if (or especially because) the products they sell are not consistent with healthy eating guidelines. A principled view might see such PPPs as inappropriately giving kudos to the manufacturer of energy-dense, nutrient-poor food products. They might also see such PPPs as being vulnerable to conflicts of interest, real or perceived. Such a situation would arise if the food fortification activity were exploited by the partner to give it special market access to sell its food products, or if it required a government to purchase its premix product to support the activity.

The management of PPPs is very much about the management of power relationships among partners. The resources available to prospective BINGO and PINGO partners can outweigh those available to sovereign nations and the UN agencies that traditionally have planned, delivered, monitored, and evaluated food fortification activities. There is a power differential in such partnerships and the consequent risk of 'institutional capture' by powerful partners (60). In this setting, it is essential that managers avoid conflicts of interest from arising, put in place safeguards to protect public health interests being co-opted by commercial interests, and avoid inappropriate sponsorship and co-branding arrangements with food and beverage products that are inconsistent with healthy eating guidelines (68).

Starting with the publication of the 1987 WHO document: 'Principles governing relations between the World Health Organization and nongovernmental organizations', that was adopted by the 40th WHA, 1987, resolution WHA40.25 (69), the WHO and WHA have undertaken a number of reviews, approved resolutions, and released a series of guidelines for managing potential risks and benefits associated with PPPs. In 2000, the WHO 2000 published: *Guidelines on working with the private sector to achieve health outcomes* (70), and in 2002 published its review of how it interacts with civil society and NGOs (71). Then, in 2010, the 63rd WHA approved resolution WHA 63.10 that deals with WHO involvement in partnerships (72). This WHA resolution endorsed a new policy on WHO's engagement with global health partnerships and hosting arrangements (73). The policy submitted as an annex to the resolution provides the framework that will guide WHO's assessment of, and decisions concerning, potential engagement in different types of health partnerships. It establishes criteria, including that there be added value for public health, and that potential conflicts of interest shall be taken into consideration as part of the design and structure of a prospective partnership with commercial, for-profit companies. The resolution also requested the director-general to continue collaboration with several partners, including private sector entities, in implementing the WHO medium-term strategic plan 2008–2013.

Conclusion

Food fortification policies and regulations are formulated within national and global food regulatory systems. These systems manage political debates associated with food fortification and in particular the contrasting public health and commercial objectives for investing in this technology. Food fortification politics is played out through the engagement of actors with food regulatory systems, is expressed through the activities of these actors, and is influenced by the dominant underpinning agendas within which food regulatory systems operate.

Two characteristics of the food fortification actors and their activities stand out, especially at the global food regulatory system level. First is the substantial number of actors involved with an interest in expanding and promoting food fortification as a technology for supporting public health and/or commercial interests. Most actors that engage with food regulatory systems tend to be well-resourced and organized to act as professional entities that represent a particular interest. They have power in framing food regulatory system agendas, influencing decision-making and shaping outcomes. Actors may dispute the reason for or details of certain food fortification activities, but few, if any, actors explicitly oppose the concept of food fortification, if they do exist they are not highly visible. Second is the degree of interaction among these powerful actors. Many actors act in coalitions, alliances, and partnerships to secure food fortification outcomes that support their interests. There is less evidence that individual citizens are significantly engaged with or directly represented in food regulatory systems. Instead they are passive recipients of food fortification regulation outcomes that manifest in their exposure to novel composition profiles of certain food products.

Several dominant political agendas are influencing food fortification governance arrangements and in turn this is influencing actors and the activities they undertake. Both at national and global levels there is an ideological agenda shaping the relative power and roles of the public, private, and civil society sectors when participating in food fortification activities. An investment in new management system approaches is characterized by a deregulation agenda and the pursuit of greater private and civil sector involvement in food fortification policies and programmes. Food regulatory systems are changing their decision-making tools so as to reduce barriers to those actors seeking food product innovations. There is increasing participation by transnational actors such as BINGOs and PINGOs in intergovernmental organizations such as WHO and UNICEF. They have significant influence over the development and implementation of food fortification policies and programmes, activities that traditionally have been under the purview of the state. In addition, the delineation between national and global food regulatory systems is becoming less pronounced. National government food regulation arrangements increasingly are being influenced by global health governance arrangements because of global food trade and the consequent drive towards international harmonization of food policies and regulations.

The influence of the actors, their activities, and the dominant agendas on food fortification activities was analysed in each of the case studies presented in Section 2 of this book. In the next chapter, the approach that was used to investigate these case studies is described. It is informed by the earlier review of relevant policy science theoretical frameworks to help gain insights to explain how and why evidence, ethics, and politics interact in food fortification activities.

References

1. Sommer A. How public health policy is created: scientific process and political reality. *American Journal of Epidemiology* 2001; 154(12 Suppl):S4–6.
2. Lang T, Heasman M. *Food wars. The global battle for mouths, minds and markets.* London: Earthscan; 2004.

3. Nestle M. *Food politics: How the food industry influences nutrition and health.* Berkley, CA: University of California Press; 2002.

4. Walt G. *Health policy: an introduction to process and power.* Johannesburg: Witwatersrand University Press; 1994.

5. US Department of Agriculture. Global Food Markets: Global Food Industry Structure. Economic Research Center, US Department of Agriculture; 2011. [cited 26 September 2012]. Available from: http://www.ers.usda.gov/Briefing/GlobalFoodMarkets/Industry.htm.

6. Liese A. Explaining varying degrees of openness in the Food and Agriculture Organization of the United Nations. In: Jönsson C, Tallberg, J. (eds). *Transnational actors in global governance: patterns, explanations and implications.* Basingstoke: Palgrave Macmillan; 2010, pp. 88–108.

7. Laswell H. *Politics: who gets what, when, how.* New York: McGraw-Hill; 1936.

8. Allen L, de Benoist B, Dary O, Hurrell R. *Guidelines on food fortification with micronutrients.* Geneva: World Health Organization; 2006. Available from: http://www.who.int/nutrition/publications/guide_food_fortification_micronutrients.pdf.

9. Rein M, Schön D. Reframing policy discourse. In: Fischer F, Forester J, (eds). *The Argumentative Turn in Policy Analysis and Planning.* London: Duke University Press; 1993. pp. 145–66.

10. Food Standards Agency. [cited 23 December 2011]. Available from: http://www.food.gov.uk/foodindustry/regulation/betregs/#top.

11. Australian Department of Finance and Deregulation, Office of Best Practice Regulation. *Best practice regulation handbook, 2010.* Canberra: 2010.

12. Cabinet Office. *Food matters: Towards a strategy for the 21st century.* London: Cabinet Office; 2008.

13. World Trade Organization. *Agreement on technical barriers to trade.* [cited 27 March 2012]. Available from: http://www.wto.org/english/res_e/booksp_e/analytic_index_e/tbt_01_e.htm.

14. Lawrence M. *Using domestic law in the fight against obesity: an introductory guide for the Pacific.* World Health Organization: Geneva; 2003.

15. World Health Organization/World Trade Organization. *WTO agreements and public health: A joint study by the WHO and the WTO secretariat.* World Health Organization: Geneva; 2002.

16. Darnton-Hill I, Nalubola R. Fortification strategies to meet micronutrient needs: successes and failures. *Proceedings of The Nutrition Society* 2002; 61(2): 231–41.

17. Codex Alimentarius Commission. [cited 3 February 2012]. Available from: http://www.codexalimentarius.org.

18. Codex Alimentarius Commission. *Codex Alimentarius Commission, Procedural Manual.* Geneva: Food and Agriculture Organization of the United Nations/World Health Organization; 2011.

19. Codex Alimentarius Commission. Understanding codex [cited 3 February 2012]. Available from: http://www.codexalimentarius.org/about-codex/understanding-codex/en/.

20. Food and Agriculture Organization/World Health Organization. *Understanding the Codex Alimentarius.* Geneva: Food and Agriculture Organization/World Health Organization; 2006.

21. Codex Alimentarius Commission. *General principles for the addition of essential nutrients to foods (CAC/GL 09-1987, amended 1989, 1991)*. Geneva: Food and Agriculture Organization/World Health Organization; 1987.

22. Codex Alimentarius Commission. *Codex committee on nutrition and foods for special dietary uses, thirty first session*. Geneva: Food and Agriculture Organization/World Health Organization; 2009.

23. Codex Committee on Nutrition and Foods for Special Dietary Uses, CX/NFSDU 12/34/9 (Agenda Item 6), Proposed draft revision of the Codex General Principles for the addition of essential nutrients to foods (CAC/GL 9-1987). Germany; 3–7 December 2012.

24. Food and Agriculture Organization. [cited 28 March 2012]. Available from: http://www.fao.org/.

25. Food and Agriculture Organization. *Policy statement: fortification of food with micronutrients*. [cited 28 March 2012]. Available from: ftp://ftp.fao.org/docrep/fao/005/y8346m/y8346m10.pdf.

26. United Nations International Children's Emergency Fund. [cited 28 March 2012]. Available from: www.unicef.org.

27. World Food Programme. *How WFP fights malnutrition*. [cited 4 April 2012]. Available from: http://www.wfp.org/nutrition/how-wfp-fights-malnutrition.

28. World Health Organization. *Nutrition*. [cited 27 March 2012]. Available from: http://www.who.int/nutrition/about_us/en/.

29. World Health Organization. *Vitamin and Mineral Nutrition Information System (VMNIS)*. [cited 2 December 2011]. Available from: http://www.who.int/vmnis/about/en/.

30. World Health Organization. *Recommendations on wheat and maize flour fortification meeting report: interim consensus statement*. Geneva: World Health Organization; 2009 [cited 28 March 2012]. Available from: http://www.who.int/nutrition/publications/micronutrients/wheat_maize_fortification/en/index.html.

31. World Health Organization. *Electronic library of evidence for nutrition actions (eLENA)*. [cited 28 March 2012]. Available from: http://www.who.int/elena/en/index.html.

32. International Food Policy Research Institute. *About IFPRI*. [cited 29 March 2012]. Available from: http://www.ifpri.org/ourwork/about.

33. Harvest Plus. [cited 3 June 2012]. Available from: http://www.harvestplus.org.

34. US Agency for International Development. [cited 23 March 2012]. Available from: http://www.usaid.gov.

35. The World Bank. [cited 3 June 2012]. Available from: http://www.worldbank.org.

36. The World Bank. *Enriching lives: overcoming vitamin and mineral malnutrition in developing countries*. Washington, DC: The World Bank; 1994.

37. Micronutrient Initiative. *Micronutrient Initiative five-year strategic plan 2008–2013*. [cited 3 April 2012]. Available from: http://www.micronutrient.org/CMFiles/What%20we%20do/Vision%20-%20Purpose%20-%20Mission/strategicplan.pdf.

38. Micronutrient Initiative. *2010–2011 annual report*. [cited 3 April 2012]. Available from: http://www.micronutrient.org/CMFiles/MI-AnnualReport1011-EN-web.pdf.

39. Sight and Life. [cited 2012 3 April]. Available from: http://www.sightandlife.org/.

40. DSM Nutritional Products. [cited 3 June 2012]. Available from: www.dsmnutritionalproducts.com.

41. Bill and Melinda Gates Foundation. *Foundation fact sheet.* [cited 3 April 2012]. Available from: http://www.gatesfoundation.org/about/Pages/foundation-fact-sheet.aspx.

42. Gates B. *UNICEF and the Micronutrient Initiative.* [cited 23 January 2012]. Available from: http://www.unicef.org/china/VMD_for_Food_Industry_in_English_-_25_August.pdf.

43. World Health Organization. *Public–private partnerships for health 2011* [cited 20 March 2012]. Available from: http://www.who.int/trade/glossary/story077/en/index.html.

44. Global Alliance for Improved Nutrition. *Business alliance.* 2009 [cited November 2010]. Available from: http://www.gainhealth.org/partnerships/business-alliance.

45. Global Alliance for Improved Nutrition (ed). *Partnerships and collaboration. Summary of the workshop. Business seeking solutions to the fight against malnutrition. 4th GAIN Business Alliance Forum 25–26 May*; 2010; Dubai, United Arab Emirates.

46. Global Alliance for Improved Nutrition. *About GAIN.* 2011 [cited 23 March 2012]. Available from: http://www.gainhealth.org/about-gain.

47. Carriere R. Public-private sector alliances for food fortification: time for optimism. *Food and Nutrition Bulletin* 2003; 24(4 Suppl):S155–9.

48. Bekefi T. *Micronutrient deficiency and the global alliance for improved nutrition: lessons in multisectoral partnership.* Cambridge, MA: John F. Kennedy School of Government, Harvard University; 2006. Available from: http://www.hks.harvard.edu/m-rcbg/CSRI/publications/report_7_Bekefi_micronutrient_2006FNL1-23-07.pdf.

49. Nutraingredients. *New funding for vitamin-enriched foods in Asia.* [cited 16 September 2011]. Available from: http://www.nutraingredients.com/Industry/New-funding-for-vitamin-enriched-foods-in-Asia.

50. Flour Fortification Initiative. *Public-private-civic investment in each nation.* [cited 19 March 2012]. Available from: http://www.sph.emory.edu/wheatflour/index.php.

51. Flour Fortification Initiative. [cited 19 March 2012]. Available from: http://www.sph.emory.edu/wheatflour/strategy.php.

52. McLachlan M, Garrett J. Nutrition change strategies: the new frontier. *Public Health Nutrition* 2008; 11(10):1063–75.

53. World Health Organization. *Global health partnerships: progress on developing draft policy guidelines for WHO's involvement.* Report by the Secretariat. Executive Board. 123rd Session. EB 123/6. 18 April 2008 [cited July 2011]. Available from: http://apps.who.int/gb/ebwha/pdf_files/EB123/B123_6-en.pdf.

54. United Nations System Standing Committee on Nutrition. *Scaling Up Nutrition: A Framework for Action. Based on a series of consultations hosted by the Center for Global Development, the International Conference on Nutrition.* USAID, UNICEF and the World Bank; 2010.

55. Tallberg J, Jönsson C. Transnational actor participation in international institutions: where, why, and with what consequences? In: Jönsson C, Tallberg J (eds). *Transnational actors in global governance: patterns, explanations and implications.* Basingstoke: Palgrave Macmillan; 2010. pp. 1–21.

56. United Nations International Children's Emergency Fund. *Vitamins & minerals for children fortifies economic development in China.* [cited 23 January 2012]. Available from: http://www.unicef.org/media/media_23416.html.

57. United Nations International Children's Emergency Fund and the Micronutrient Initiative. *Vitamin and mineral deficiency: a challenge to the world's food companies.* 2004 [cited 24 January 2012]. Available from: http://www.micronutrient.org/CMFiles/PubLib/Report-70-VMD-A-chanllenge-to-the-Worlds-Food-Companies1NMP-3242008-7366.pdf.

58. Zammit A, Utting P. *Beyond pragmatism: appraising UN-business partnerships.* Paper No. 1. PP-MBR-1. Geneva: United Nations Research Institute for Social Development; 2006. Available from: http://www.unrisd.org/80256B3C005BCCF9/(httpPublications)/225508544695E8F3C12572300038ED22?.

59. World Health Organization, editor. *Health development in a changing world—a call for action, resolution WHA46.17, WHA46/1993/REC/1.* Forty-sixth World Health Assembly, 3–14 May 1993. Geneva: World Health Organization; 1993.

60. Buse K, Waxman A. Public–private health partnerships: a strategy for WHO. *Bulletin of the World Health Organization* 2001; 79:748–54.

61. United Nations. Keeping the promise: a forward-looking review to promote an agreed action agenda to achieve the Millennium Development Goals by 2015. Report of the Secretary-General. [cited 3 June 2012]. Available from: http://www.un.org/ga/search/view_doc.asp?symbol=A/64/665&referer=http://www.unscn.org/admin/modules_edit.php?module=6&Lang=E.

62. Mannar M, van Ameringen M. Role of public-private partnership in micronutrient food fortification. *Food and Nutrition Bulletin* 2003; 24(4 Suppl):S151–4.

63. World Health Organization. *Micronutrients evidence-informed guideline.* [cited 22 March 2012]. Available from: http://www.who.int/nutrition/publications/micronutrients/guidelines/en/index.html.

64. Brady M, Rundall P. Governments should govern, and corporations should follow the rules. In: *SCN News. Nutrition and Business: How to Engage?* No. 39 late 2011. Available from: http://www.unscn.org/files/Publications/SCN_News/SCNNEWS39_10.01_high_def.pdf.

65. Buse K, Harmer A. Seven habits of highly effective global public-private health partnerships: practice and potential. *Social Science and Medicine* 2007; 64(2):259–71.

66. Hawkes C, Buse K. Public health sector and food industry interaction: it's time to clarify the term 'partnership' and be honest about underlying interests. *European Journal of Public Health* 2011; 21(4):400–1.

67. Zimmerman R. Gates fights malnutrition with cheese, ketchup incentives. *Wall Street Journal.* 2002; Sect. B.1–B.

68. Richter J. *Public-private partnerships and international health policy-making: how can public interests be safeguarded?* Geneva: World Health Organization/Virot, P; 2004 [cited June 2011]. Available from: http://formin.finland.fi/public/download.aspx?ID=12360&GUID={3556FE5F-6CBC-4000-86F3-99EBFD2778FC.

69. World Health Organization. *Fortieth World Health Assembly, 1987, resolution WHA40.25.* Geneva: World Health Organization; 2001.

70. World Health Organization. *Guidelines on working with the private sector to achieve health outcomes. Executive board 107th Session. EB107/20, 30 November 2000* [cited 22 March 2012]. Available from: http://apps.who.int/gb/archive/pdf_files/EB107/ee20.pdf.

71. World Health Organization. *WHO's Interactions with civil society and nongovernmental organizations. Civil society initiative. External relations and governing bodies.* Geneva: World Health Organization; 2002 [cited 22 March 2012]. Available from: http://www. who.int/civilsociety/documents/en/RevreportE.pdf.

72. World Health Assembly. *Sixty-third World Health Assembly, WHA63.10. Partnerships. Resolutions and decisions.* Geneva: World Health Organization; 2010.

73. World Health Assembly. *Sixty-third World Health Assembly, WHA63.10. Partnerships. Agenda item 18.1. 21.* Geneva: World Health Organization; 2010.

Chapter 4

Investigating food fortification

> . . . public policy and the problems with which it is concerned do not exist in neat, tidy, academic boxes . . . the aim of the policy approach is not to pull these issues apart, so much as to recognize how problems come to be addressed and structured by the way in which knowledge is organized and deployed . . . consequently and inevitably the study of policy-making and policy analysis is essentially multiframed (1).

> (Reproduced with permission from Parsons W, Public policy: an introduction to the theory and practice of policy analysis, Cheltenham, Edward Elgar Publishing Ltd, Copyright ©1995.)

Introduction

The investigation of food fortification as a technological intervention to tackle problems associated with inadequate nutrient intakes is an especially challenging policy research topic. As outlined in previous chapters, evidence and ethics inform food fortification policy-making often through non-rational processes and, as this is a highly contested topic, politics inevitably is omnipresent in food fortification activities. These challenges are set against the context of there being a variety of underlying causes of inadequate nutrient intakes and potentially many different policy solutions available to address the resulting policy problems. An innovative research approach from within the discipline of political science was required to achieve the research aim of providing insights into and understandings of food fortification policy-making, so as to help practitioners identify how existing policy processes and outcomes might be improved to further protect and promote public health.

A multi-framed policy science approach was needed so that the investigation moved beyond measuring and evaluating a policy's impact and instead analysed antecedent policy-making processes (2). This food fortification investigation was predicated on the policy science notion that 'facts' are value-laden and that the translation of evidence into food fortification policy is inherently political. Therefore an understanding of food fortification policy-making requires recognizing the interplay between political variables and evidence-informed policy practice.

The present investigation invoked Walt and her colleagues' recommendation that in undertaking policy analysis, researchers need to use existing frameworks and theories of the public policy process and make research design an explicit concern in their studies (3). The frameworks and theories presented in Chapters 2 and 3 were used to guide the assessment and analysis of each of the case studies and help provide answers to this investigation's research questions. The assessment component of each case study was based on the evidence available for public health benefits, risks, and ethical considerations of each policy intervention. The way that evidence and ethical justifications were used in the policy-making process for each case study was then analysed to help explain how and why policies are made. This chapter provides a description of the case study research design and methods conducted in undertaking the policy analysis for this investigation.

The research design

The research design for this investigation had two inter-related components: assessment and analysis. First, the assessment component set up the investigation to answer research question 1, i.e. 'What are the public health benefits, risks, and ethical considerations of food fortification?'. The findings from the first component informed the second, the analytical component that set up the investigation to answer research question 2, i.e. 'How and why are food fortification policies made?'. This is because in analysing how and why food fortification policy is made, it was necessary to know what other policy interventions are available and how they and food fortification perform against evidential and ethical evaluative frameworks. For instance, a food fortification intervention assessed as performing poorly against evaluative frameworks relative to alternative policy interventions yet is implemented as the preferred intervention, raises different analytical questions to the situation in which a food fortification intervention performs impressively and was the preferred intervention.

The case study research design and methods proposed by Yin (4) were adapted for this investigation. Case study research is in-depth empirical inquiry into phenomena in their real-life context. This research method possesses distinctive qualities that are especially suited to: answering 'how' and 'why' research questions, and analysing topics where the focus is on contemporary events and circumstances where the investigator has no control over those events. Case studies can be exploratory, descriptive, or explanatory. The case study research for this investigation extended beyond exploration to obtain data that were assessed and analysed to describe evidence-informed food fortification policy-making.

Food fortification policy is not a homogenous entity. A substantial number of food fortification interventions with different rationales and involving different combinations of nutrients and food vehicles are available for interrogation. In this book's introduction chapter, three distinct public health rationales for increasing the intake of a nutrient were identified and each linked to a policy problem for which food fortification was a potential policy solution.

The research design for this investigation was a single-case study design applied to each of these three rationales to assess public health benefits, risks, and ethical considerations associated with food fortification and to analyse how and why food fortification policies are made. According to Yin (4), a single-case study design can be a legitimate approach to gain theoretical understandings if it is a *representative* case that captures the typical circumstances and conditions of the phenomenon under investigation. The aim of this research design was to achieve a comprehensive assessment and analysis of food fortification and its policy-making processes. In this investigation the observations from each of the three case studies were compared with each of the other case studies to identify further patterns to help explain collectively how and why food fortification policy is made. The justification for the selection of the three case studies is that they each are a representative case of one of the following three identified rationales for food fortification:

1 Universal salt iodization to help prevent iodine deficiency disorders is the representative case when food fortification is proposed as a policy response to an inadequate amount of a nutrient, or combination of nutrients, available from the food supply.

2 Mandatory flour fortification with folic acid to help reduce the risk of neural tube defects is the representative case when food fortification is proposed as a policy response to the presence of a medical condition that results in a need for a raised nutrient intake in certain at-risk individuals.

3 Mandatory milk fortification with vitamin D to help prevent vitamin D deficiency is the representative case when food fortification is proposed as a policy response to a reduction in the primary source of a nutrient.

Research method for assessing each case study

The research method for assessing each case study was based on the premise that when planning a food fortification policy, policy-makers are invariably confronted with evidential challenges and ethical considerations. From an evidential perspective they often need to make decisions in the context of incomplete evidence and/or uncertainties about benefits and risks associated with the relationship. From an ethical perspective a food fortification policy often has consequences related to its impact on an individual's and the collective's rights and needs.

When policy-makers assess the appropriateness of a food fortification policy intervention to respond to evidence of a policy problem, there are three evidence- and ethics-related questions that arise:

1 How to specify and measure public health benefits and risks?

2 How to specify and measure the ethical considerations?

3 How to compare the scientific uncertainties and ethical considerations across the possible policy solutions available?

Each case study was assessed to identify and describe the public health benefits, risks, and ethical considerations of the food fortification intervention and thereby help answer research question 1: 'What are the public health benefits, risks, and ethical considerations associated with food fortification?'.

Many health authorities, including the World Health Organization, have adopted evidence-based practice as the primary system for assessing the public health case for, and impact of, food fortification. Others argue that ethical principles should underpin policy-making associated with public health interventions such as food fortification and then evidence and theory should help inform aspects of decision-making (5). This investigation adopts the view taken by Carter et al. (6) that evidence and ethics are implicitly related, e.g. evidence-based practice may be more ethical, and ethically sensitive practice more effective, and as such they are assessed together iteratively.

Data collection

Epidemiological and aetiological evidence to inform the background to each case study, as well as evaluative evidence to inform the assessment of its public health benefits, risks, and ethical considerations (and that of alternative policy options), was obtained from desk-based research of the scientific literature and presented as a narrative review.

Data assessment

The assessment of each case study took place in two stages. First, the background to the health concern related to the case study was described. Second, the public health benefits, risks, and ethical considerations were assessed and compared. Public health benefits were assessed in relation to four criteria: evidence of effectiveness, cost-effectiveness, equity, and practical advantages of the policy option. Public health risks were assessed in relation to primary public health risk (evidence of the potential for acute safety concerns associated with excessive nutrient intake), secondary public health risk (evidence of chronic public health concerns associated with the potential to distort dietary intakes and promote dietary imbalances), and practical disadvantages of a particular intervention. The assessment of ethical considerations involved assessing how closely the policy solution adhered to each of the five 'justificatory conditions': effectiveness, proportionality, necessity, least infringement, and public justification, proposed by Childress et al. (7) (Chapter 2).

Food fortification is just one among many policy interventions that may have a role in preventing and controlling inadequate nutrient intakes. As Allen et al. comment:

> Fortification of food with micronutrients is a valid technology for reducing micronutrient malnutrition as part of a food-based approach when and where existing food supplies and limited access fail to provide adequate levels of the respective nutrients in the diet. In such cases, food fortification reinforces and supports ongoing nutrition improvement programmes and should be regarded as part of a broader, integrated approach to prevent MNM [micronutrient malnutrition], thereby complementing other approaches to improve micronutrient status (8).

It is an ethical principle that the public health benefits, risks, and ethical considerations of food fortification policy interventions should be assessed against plausible alternative policy solutions to policy problems. For each case study the assessment was conducted on the food fortification intervention itself, as well as for plausible alternative policy solutions to enable an assessment comparison to be made. The options that were identified as plausible alternative policy solutions to food fortification for the three policy problems are drawn from one or more of the following:

♦ Supplementation: supplementation refers to promoting the consumption of a 'dose' of a micronutrient usually available in pill, capsule, or supplement form. The micronutrient dosage can be tightly controlled and its delivery highly targeted to specific individuals and population groups. It can have a rapid impact on the nutrient status of consumers.

♦ Public health, social, and agricultural development measures: in this investigation public health measures is a broad descriptor to capture a diversity of policy options that vary with the nature of the policy problem being addressed. Common public health measures in helping tackle micronutrient malnutrition are: improvements in water sanitation, intestinal parasite control, and control of infectious diseases (9). In addition there are a number of measures that aim to tackle underpinning structural causes of hunger and micronutrient malnutrition. Examples of such measures are social development activities to help alleviate poverty and activities to help reform food an agricultural systems to support the production of local micronutrient-rich foods. For the mandatory milk fortification with vitamin D case study the promotion of sunlight exposure is categorized as a public health measure.

◆ Nutrition education: nutrition education in this context refers to both a message content and a message delivery process. The message content focuses on the importance of dietary diversification and healthy eating and lifestyle principles such as promoting breastfeeding. The message delivery process ranges from relatively passive activities, such as social marketing campaigns and information material distributed as leaflets or posters, through to more interactive education opportunities to strengthen knowledge, problem solving, and skills development to help change dietary behaviour. Nutrition education is a relatively 'soft' policy option as it is not particularly costly or politically risky for governments, and instead much of the onus to put the education into practice is left to individuals and the general public.

A secondary focus for nutrition education is to inform people about the policy problem and various policy interventions as well as to inform health practitioners who are critical for putting the policy interventions into practice.

◆ Maintaining the status quo: maintaining the status quo means that no explicit policy intervention is undertaken to address evidence of an existing problem. This may be because a conscious decision is made not to intervene, e.g. the decision is that a precautionary approach to the policy problem is warranted. Alternatively it might be because no decision is made and the status quo option reflects lack of attention to the policy problem for a variety of potential reasons such as lack of interest, capacity, resources, and/or awareness of the policy problem. This option includes stopping an existing policy intervention that is addressing the policy problem.

The ideal policy response may be a combination of policy options in a multi-pronged strategy with the relative importance of particular options depending on local circumstances. For example, Darnton-Hill explains how interventions such as supplementation are short-term measures, whereas food-based approaches (including food fortification) are a medium-term approach, while related public health interventions tend to be more longer term (10). For the purposes of this investigation, each of these policy options was assessed as a standalone intervention and in generic terms, i.e. it was assumed that the policy problem was prevalent in a particular country. Although this is the only feasible approach to manage the assessment of interventions, it is acknowledged that this does not necessarily reflect the ideal approach for implementing interventions in practice. Often the best and most sustainable approach for effectively and sustainably addressing inadequate nutrient intakes is to have a combination of interventions implemented as complementary, mutually reinforcing strategies. In addition, the relative importance of a particular intervention will be influenced by local circumstances and needs, e.g. the level of prevalence of a policy problem in a country.

Research method for analysing each case study

The research method for analysing each case study was informed by policy science theories. The review of theories and models of evidence-informed policy-making (Chapter 3) revealed the powerful role of actors, their activities, and underlying agendas in influencing the policy-making process. The method was concerned with capturing processes and studying real-world situations as they unfolded naturally, it was non-manipulative and open to whatever emerged with a lack of predetermined constraints on outcomes. It used a naturalistic approach to inductively and holistically understand food fortification policy-making processes. With a holistic perspective the whole phenomenon under study (food fortification policy-making) was understood as a complex system that is more than the sum of its parts and the focus of inquiry was on investigating complex interactions within the system (11). In this investigation, case studies were 'deconstructed' to expose interactions between the actors, their activities, and the underlying agendas with evidence and ethics. They were then 'reconstructed' to provide the most plausible description of the use of evidence and ethics in the making of the food fortification intervention represented in each case study and thereby help answer research question 2: 'How and why are food fortification policies made?'

Data collection

Food fortification policy-related documents were the main data source for the case study inquiries. The sources searched for the more significant and relevant documents associated with each case study were: scientific publications and official documentation available in the public domain, e.g. policy documents, media releases, speeches, government, non-governmental organization, and industry reports, and newspaper clippings. The data collection focused on the more prominent documentary data sources. Data obtained from these documentary sources were used to outline the issues, the sequence of events, the processes, the actors, the activities, and the agendas associated with the policy-making process for each case study.

The quality and comprehensiveness of the data collection process for documentary sources is vulnerable to the potential for selectivity in those documents made available for retrieval and reporting bias within the document.

It cannot be assumed that all documentation associated with a case study was available or accessible or that those documents that were collected provided a comprehensive, accurate, and unbiased record of events. Indeed, the more revealing, and potentially more sensitive documented accounts of the policy-making processes are often those that are more difficult to access. Several approaches to achieve as comprehensive coverage of relevant documents as possible were implemented. The collection of documents was an iterative process. The information contained in certain documents led to the identification of information gaps and the existence of, or need to locate, additional documents. All collected documents were read.

Data analysis

Policy rarely occurs at one point in time. The collected data were presented chronologically, structured as a narrative organized around the primary milestones, actors, activities, and underpinning agendas in the case study's history, to make sense of how and why each case study was made. The data mostly illustrate global developments with some national examples included where relevant.

In acknowledging the critiques of the stages heuristic model of policy-making (Chapter 3), organizing the data in this way was not to suggest that all policy processes and debates were discrete and chronological. Instead a time-line structure enabled the case study to be deconstructed and processes and policy debates to be viewed as they unfolded over time. The data were analysed to identify the presence and influence of actors, activities, and agendas during the policy process for each case study narrative by asking the following sets of questions:

1 Actors

  ◆ Who are the actors associated with each case study?

  ◆ What are their views about the policy problem and available policy solutions?

  ◆ What resources and capacity do they have available?

2 Activities (advocacy and the framing of the policy problem and the policy solution)

As policy analysis has shifted from rational models to more interpretive models, a focus on analysing advocacy and framing activities has been recommended to help explain how policy-makers construct problems and structure policy action (12). Framing refers to the processes of meaning and legitimation given to a policy problem and the policy response, how agendas are set and problems conceived. The policy analysis approach used in this research involved exposing often hidden contested values, beliefs, and interests that are captured when representing a policy problem and solution in a certain way using the following questions:

- How was the policy problem represented?
- Who was responsible for this representation?
- Who benefits from this representation?
- What policy solutions were/are offered?
- How do these solutions represent the issue?
- What assumptions underlie this representation?
- What aspects of the issue were/are not considered?

3 Agendas

- What, if any, was the influence of dominant political ideologies on policy processes?
- What, if any, was the influence of global food trade and international obligations on policy processes?
- What, if any, was the influence of global health governance and the pursuit of public-private partnerships on policy processes?

Because the investigation focused mostly on global level data and the use of food fortification as a public health intervention, it was the global health governance agenda that was especially relevant to the case study analyses.

An interpretive approach was applied to identify the various values, beliefs, and interests in the representation of a policy problem and solution. In this way it was possible to investigate, in the course of the interplay among the three policy variables, how the policy problem was defined and represented, and how different policy solutions were represented, promoted and/or hidden. In addition, this investigation used a framing approach to study the meanings given to the policy problems, causes, and solutions emerging from the interactions among actors, activities, and agendas during the policy identification and implementation process. Problem framing refers to how different actors often have different ways of thinking about a problem, and their various perspectives are enmeshed in the way they define, present, and examine that problem. This can affect how concepts like aetiology and causality are discussed and researched. The interactions were interpreted against theoretical frameworks to construct the most plausible description of the use of evidence and ethics in each case study. The descriptions obtained for each of the three case studies then were combined to generate an understandable and experientially credible description of food fortification policy-making overall.

While statistical generalization and establishing causal relationships cannot be addressed using a case study, analytical generalization (expanding and generalizing theoretical propositions) can be achieved (4). The frame of reference for this research was food fortification as a technology for public health nutrition policy (this is the level to which the study findings are generalized).

Conclusion

Values, beliefs, and interests typically shape views towards the relationships between food and health, including how such relationships should be studied and the utility of the evidence for such relationships for informing food fortification policy. Moral views determine what ought to happen where tensions exist between the common good and the need to protect individual rights. Differences in values, beliefs, and interests create a fertile setting for politics to exert influence over how and why evidence and ethics are interpreted and applied in food fortification policy-making. The case study research design and methods that are used in this investigation were selected for their ability to reveal such dynamics and help describe how and why they happen in practice. In the next three chapters, food fortification case studies based on different rationales for food fortification policy are critically assessed and analysed.

References

1. Parsons W. *Public policy: an introduction to the theory and practice of policy analysis.* Cheltenham: Edward Elgar Publishing Ltd; 1995.
2. Bernier N, Clavier C. Public health policy research: making the case for a political science approach. *Health Promotion International* 2011; 26(1):109–16.
3. Walt G, Shiffman, J, Schneider, H, Murray, SF, Brugha, R, Gilson, L. 'Doing' health policy analysis: methodological and conceptual reflections and challenges. *Health Policy and Planning* 2008; 23(5):308–17.
4. Yin R. *Case study research: design and methods*, 4th ed. Thousand Oaks, CA: Sage Publications; 2009.
5. Tannahill A. Beyond evidence—to ethics: a decision-making framework for health promotion, public health and health improvement. *Health Promotion International* 2008; 23(4):380–90.
6. Carter S, Rychetnik L, Lloyd B, Kerridge I, Baur L, Bauman A, *et al.* Evidence, ethics, and values: a framework for health promotion. *American Journal of Public Health* 2011; 101(3):465–72.
7. Childress J, Faden R, Gaare R, Gostin L, Kahn J, Bonnie R, *et al.* Public health ethics: mapping the terrain. *Journal of Law, Medicine and Ethics* 2002; 30(2):170–8.
8. Allen L, de Benoist B, Dary O, Hurrell R. *Guidelines on food fortification with micronutrients.* Geneva: World Health Organization; 2006 [cited 25 September 2012]; Available from: http://www.who.int/nutrition/publications/guide_food_fortification_micronutrients.pdf.
9. Howson C, Kennedy E, Horwitz A (eds). *Prevention of micronutrient deficiencies: tools for policy makers and public health workers.* Washington, DC: National Academy Press; 1998.

10. Darnton-Hill I. Control and prevention of micronutrient malnutrition. *Asia Pacific Journal of Clinical Nutrition* 1998; 7(1):2–7.

11. Patton M. *Qualitative evaluation and research methods*. Newbury Park, CA: Sage; 1990.

12. Godin B. *The making of science, technology and innovation policy: conceptual frameworks as narratives, 1945-2005*. Montreal: Centre Urbanisation Culture Société; 2009.

Section 2

The case studies

This section of the book presents the case studies for the investigation. Food fortification is a broad topic and there are many policy interventions underway. Three case studies were selected to collectively represent all potential rationales for mandatory food fortification as an intervention to protect and promote public health. These case studies and the particular public health rationale that they are representing are:

Case study 1: universal salt iodization as an intervention to help prevent iodine deficiency disorders

Universal salt iodization was selected as the representative case for assessing and analysing the use of mandatory food fortification as a policy solution for policy problems that arise when the food supply is unable to provide sufficient nutrients for health.

Case study 2: mandatory flour fortification with folic acid to help reduce the risk of neural tube defects

Mandatory flour fortification with folic acid was selected as the representative case for assessing and analysing the use of mandatory food fortification as a policy solution for policy problems that arise when certain individuals have nutrient requirements higher than reference standards.

Case study 3: mandatory milk fortification with vitamin D to help prevent vitamin D deficiency

Mandatory milk fortification with vitamin D was selected as the representative case for assessing and analysing the use of mandatory food fortification as a policy solution for policy problems that arise when there is a reduction in exposure to the primary source of a nutrient.

For each individual case study, the evidence-informed public health benefits and risks as well as the ethical considerations, are assessed and compared with alternative potential policy solutions and the policy-making process is critically analysed. Collectively, this second section of the book illustrates a research approach that is based on a single-case study design applied three times, so that all three of the identified public health rationales for food fortification (Chapter 1) are addressed. The collective findings from each case study can be combined to help provide insights into those circumstances where mandatory food fortification is (and is not) indicated as well as providing lessons for food fortification policy and practice in total.

Chapter 5

Case study 1: universal salt iodization

A spectacularly simple, universally effective, wildly attractive and incredibly cheap technical weapon—that's iodized salt! (1).

(World Health Organization. Micronutrient deficiencies. Iodine deficiency disorders. [cited 12 April 2012]. Available from: http://www.who.int/nutrition/topics/idd/en/)

Introduction

A food supply that provides a sufficient amount and variety of vitamins and minerals for a nutritionally adequate diet is essential for optimal growth and development of children and for the maintenance of the health of adults. Conversely, if a food supply cannot provide for an adequate micronutrient intake, then this can result in conditions such as anaemia, blindness, retarded growth, poor mental development, and, ultimately, increased risk of morbidity and mortality (1–5). From a social and economic perspective, micronutrient deficiencies can impact significantly and negatively on development at the individual, community, and national levels (6).

It is over 20 years since the World Health Assembly (WHA) passed a resolution and decision on the need to take action to address micronutrient malnutrition (7). Yet, currently it is estimated that there are approximately two billion people worldwide whose diet lacks sufficient amounts of vitamins and minerals essential for health (8). Globally, iodine, iron, vitamin A, and zinc deficiencies are most prevalent (9).

Although micronutrient deficiencies contribute directly to severe and life-threatening diseases, they can be difficult to detect without a clinical examination and may be inadvertently ignored until it is too late to prevent their subclinical deficiency. It is for this reason that they are often referred to as 'hidden hunger' (10). Correcting micronutrient deficiencies requires interventions that extend beyond providing enough food to satisfy energy needs and prevent hunger. Interventions also need to focus on the nutritional quality of the food so that an adequate amount and variety of nutrients to avoid micronutrient deficiencies is consumed. The conventional purpose of mandatory food fortification is to increase the amount and variety of nutrients present in the food supply to help reduce the prevalence of inadequate dietary nutrient intakes that result in population wide micronutrient deficiencies and classic malnutrition diseases (11).

The United Nations (UN) millennium summit established millennium development goals (MDGs) to guide international development work to help bridge the gap between rights and reality for the world's poor by the year 2015 (Chapter 1). Food fortification to address malnutrition was identified as a strategic initiative aligned with six of the eight MDGs (12). In responding to data revealing that poor progress was being made towards the achievement of the MDGs, the Scaling Up Nutrition (SUN) multi-stakeholder initiative was launched in 2009 (13). The SUN initiative enjoys a high level of support from senior politicians in many governments, leaders of relevant UN agencies, and the World Bank, and senior executives of major foundations and leading civil society organizations. In effect it is 're-booting' much of the global policy agenda and practices towards preventing micronutrient malnutrition to help with the achievement of the MDGs. Although in its early days, SUN is successfully increasing investment in food fortification policies as part of its work programme.

The case study selected to assess and analyse mandatory food fortification as a policy solution for micronutrient malnutrition was universal salt iodization (USI). USI is defined as occurring: 'when all salt for human and animal consumption is iodized to the internationally agreed recommended levels' (14). Iodine deficiency has been described as the most common cause of preventable mental impairment worldwide and can lead to stunted growth and other developmental abnormalities (15). The purpose of USI is to prevent and control iodine deficiency.

USI was selected as the representative case study of this food fortification purpose for three particular reasons:

1 The magnitude of iodine deficiency as a global public health nutrition problem.

2 Iodine fortification of salt was the original wide-scale food fortification intervention when it was first implemented in the early 1920s in Switzerland (16) and the US (17).

3 USI has been the most effective food fortification policy globally to prevent and control a micronutrient malnutrition-related public health problem.

The purpose of this chapter is to present the findings of the investigation into the USI case study. The chapter starts by outlining the background to the case study. Then an assessment of the case study's public health benefits, risks, and ethical considerations relative to alternative policy options is presented followed by a chronology of key milestones in the making of USI policy. A discussion of the assessment findings and of the analysis of the actors, activities, and agendas surrounding the chronology to help explain how and why the policy was made, is provided. Emerging from the discussion are proposed future directions for preventing IDD. Finally the case study findings are generalised to construct lessons regarding the plausibility of the food fortification rationale that adding nutrients to food is evidence-informed and ethically justified in circumstances where the food supply is unable to provide sufficient nutrients for health.

Background
Iodine and health

The first recorded isolation of iodine was associated with the manufacture of gunpowder for Napoleon's army. In 1811, Bernard Courtois, a manufacturer of saltpeter, was extracting sodium salts from the ash of burned seaweed (kelp) using sulphuric acid in a copper vat when vapour from the mixture condensed on the vessel to form a crystal deposit. The iodide in the seaweed ashes had been oxidized to iodine (18). Progressively during the 1800s the essential role of iodine in human health became better understood. First in 1846 when Prevost and Mafoni proposed that endemic goitre was due to iodine deficiency and then at the end of the 19th century when Baumann demonstrated that the thyroid contains iodine (19).

Most of the 15–20 mg of iodine in a healthy adult body is concentrated in the thyroid gland where it is used in the synthesis of the containing hormones thyroxine and triiodothyronine (20). These thyroid hormones play an important role in the regulation of metabolic processes associated with growth, maturation, and thermogenesis. Neural tissues are particularly sensitive to these hormones during early fetal life and throughout childhood for brain and physical development. Although only a small amount of iodine is required for the production of the hormones, a regular dietary intake of iodine is necessary because the thyroid gland is not able to store iodine.

Food sources of iodine

Most foods have a low iodine content. Typically meat, bread, cereals, vegetables, fruits, and oils have an iodine content of approximately 2–3 µg/100 g (depending on the iodine content of the soil in which they are grown).

The richest food sources of iodine are milk, eggs, and foods of marine origin because marine plants and animals concentrate the iodine present in seawater.

These food sources can contain up to 80 μg/serving. Importantly, the iodine content of milk and eggs varies significantly and seasonally depending on whether cow and/or hen fodder has been fortified with iodine.

Among coastal communities living in seaweed-rich areas it has been observed that despite a lack of dietary iodine sources the population's iodine status can be adequate and this has been attributed to iodine inhalation. Indeed, about 36 centuries ago when there was no knowledge of iodine or its deficiency, the Chinese identified seaweed and burnt sea sponge for their therapeutic effects as a remedy for goitre and this remedy eventually found its way to England, where, in the mid-1700s, it was famed as the 'Coventry remedy' (18).

For many populations, the primary source of iodine is derived from foods whose iodine content has been influenced by the presence of iodine-containing compounds used in irrigation, fertilizers, livestock feed, dairy industry disinfectants, and bakery dough conditioners. For example, in South-Eastern Australia the reported re-emergence of iodine deficiency among certain populations in the 2000s has been attributed particularly to the transition from the use of iodophores as disinfectants for large, steel milk containers to non-iodine containing cleaning compounds (21). However, this explanation is questionable as the change in iodophore use occurred in the 1960s and 1970s. Reduced dietary iodine intake might be more accurately explained by recent behaviour changes away from the use of iodized salt in the home and at commercial food outlets. Either way, it is a precarious circumstance to rely on contamination from a disinfection practice to achieve the recommended dietary iodine intake.

Recommended intake levels

The World Health Organization (WHO) recommends a daily iodine intake of 90 μg for infants and children (0–5 years), 120 μg for school-age children (6–12 years), 150 μg for adolescents and adults, and 250 μg for pregnant and lactating women (14). Most healthy adults who are iodine sufficient can tolerate iodine intakes of up to 1 mg/day (22).

Nevertheless, excessive iodine intakes leading to median urinary iodine concentration (UIC) equal to or above 300 mg/L can have serious adverse health considerations. An excessive intake of iodine may induce autoimmune thyroiditis, hyperthyroidism, (sub)clinical hypothyroidism, and goitre (23). The risk of iodine toxicity from acute, excessive intake is highest among those who have experienced iodine deficiency and particularly among the elderly. Iodine-induced hyperthyroidism is of special concern because its symptoms are not specific and the problem often is overlooked yet it is an independent risk factor for coronary heart disease and can contribute to poor fetal neurodevelopment if present during pregnancy (24). The condition is transitory and usually resolves after the source of the excessive iodine exposure is withdrawn, subsequently the incidence rates revert to normal after one to ten years post-intervention (25).

Epidemiological evidence for the policy problem

There is a gradient of disease severity in response to levels of iodine deficiency. Relatively mild iodine deficiency, particularly in children, is associated with impaired development in visual motor skills, hearing, intelligence, and reduced growth, though these adverse effects of iodine deficiency can be at least partly reversed with sufficient iodine if addressed within the first years of life (26). Severe iodine deficiency leads to an enlargement of the thyroid gland, known as goitre, reduced synthesis of thyroid hormones (hypothyroidism), cretinism, decreased fertility rate, perinatal death, infant mortality, and mental retardation (24). The multiple adverse effects on growth and development are collectively termed iodine deficiency disorders (IDD). Iodine deficiency can be harmful throughout all life stages; however, it is particularly harmful during pregnancy, lactation, and early childhood when it may adversely affect brain development and growth.

Yet, the adverse health outcomes associated with moderate iodine deficiency are not clear cut. While some studies report that the maternal thyroid is able to adapt to low iodine intakes so as to meet the increased thyroid hormone requirements of pregnancy (27), it is essential that the pregnant woman has adequate stores, as even moderate deficiency can have a detrimental impact on brain development of fetuses, even in the absence of visible goitre in their mothers. Although the thyroid gland contains small amount of iodine that can be accessed during pregnancy, if a woman is iodine deficient before pregnancy she will have reduced capacity to nurture her developing fetus with a resulting deficiency in mental development.

The prevalence of iodine deficiency globally has been steadily decreasing in recent decades as a result of public health policy interventions. As of 2011, 29.8% of school-age children (SAC) globally are estimated as having insufficient iodine intakes as assessed using median UIC as the measure (28). Median UIC is the recommended indicator for assessing iodine status in populations and SAC iodine status is used as a proxy for total population iodine status because this population group can be relatively easily monitored through school based surveys (14). Extrapolation of the proportion of SAC having insufficient iodine intakes indicates that 1.88 billion people globally had inadequate iodine intakes in 2011.

The 2011 prevalence and geographical distribution profile of iodine nutrition around the world is shown in Figure 5.1. Drawing on international threshold criteria of public health importance of iodine nutrition (14), Andersson et al.

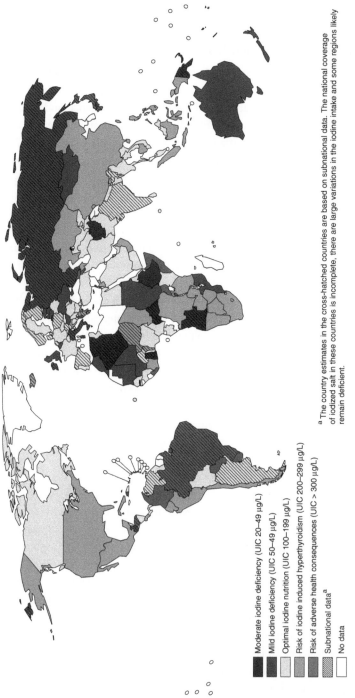

Moderate iodine deficiency (UIC 20–49 µg/L)
Mild iodine deficiency (UIC 50–49 µg/L)
Optimal iodine nutrition (UIC 100–199 µg/L)
Risk of iodine induced hyperthyroidism (UIC 200–299 µg/L)
Risk of adverse health consequences (UIC > 300 µg/L)
Subnational data[a]
No data

[a] The country estimates in the cross-hatched countries are based on subnational data. The national coverage of iodized salt in these countries is incomplete, there are large variations in the iodine intake and some regions likely remain deficient.

Fig. 5.1 Degree of public health importance of iodine nutrition in SAC based on median UIC in 2011. UIC, urinary iodine concentration; SAC, school-age children.

Andersson M et al. Global iodine status in 2011 and trends over the past decade. *The Journal of Nutrition* 142(4):744–50. Copyright © 2012 American Society for Nutrition, DOI: 10.3945/jn.111.149393.

estimated iodine intake as being inadequate (<100 mg/L) in 32 countries, adequate (100–199 mg/L) in 69, more than adequate (200–99 mg/L) in 36, and excessive (>300 mg/L) in 11(28). The figure reflects the uptake of USI and not necessarily the underlying geographical distribution of iodine-depleted soils. It illustrates that there is significant difference in the degree of iodine nutrition status in SAC around the world. The greatest proportions of children with inadequate iodine intake were in European and African regions, whereas the smallest proportions were in the Americas and the Western Pacific (28).

Cause of the policy problem

Iodine in the form of iodide is widely distributed in the earth's soils and oceans. However, it is soluble and over time is readily leached from the surface layers of soil by glaciation, flooding, and erosion. Iodine levels are particularly low in the soils of mountainous areas in China, the Andes, the Himalayas, and the European Alps. Crops grown in iodine-depleted soils contain relatively low levels of iodine and hence animal and human populations for whom a large proportion of their diets are derived from these crops are likely to be iodine deficient (20).

The geological influence on soil iodine content means that dietary iodine intake varies significantly with geography within and among countries around the world. Although most of the burden of iodine deficiency occurs in low- and middle-income countries (LMICs), many high-income countries (HICs) are not immune from this problem. It is estimated that approximately half of continental Europe is mildly iodine deficient and populations living in the inland areas of Western England and Wales, the Midwest in North America, and Southern Australia are at risk.

Multiple studies have emphasized the influence of geography and seasonality on iodine status (29–31). Observed geographical differences in clinical effects of varying iodine intake may indicate additional environmental and/or under-lying genetic variables (32, 33).

Challenges with translating the epidemiological evidence for the policy problem into a policy solution

There are two particular challenges associated with the epidemiological evidence available to inform policy and practice. First, there are the uncertainties associated with the methods for assessing the prevalence of iodine deficiency disorders. The assessment of the prevalence of iodine deficiency in populations is mainly based on UIC in SAC, which it is assumed reflect the iodine status of the general population. However, some investigators have questioned the reliability of these data and their accuracy for assessing iodine deficiency among adults, especially women of reproductive age (31, 34). In addition, the representativeness of the common approach of (sub)national sampling covering 60% of the population to estimate the number of individuals worldwide who suffer from iodine deficiency has been questioned for potentially underestimating or overestimating the extent of iodine deficiency (24).

Second, there is a lack of comprehensive monitoring of population iodine status undertaken by many countries. In 2011, 115 nationally representative country surveys were available (28). This is a significant increase over the past decade but a lack of monitoring of UIC in SAC persists in many countries.

Assessing the public health benefits, risks, and ethical considerations of policy options

The epidemiological evidence for the iodine deficiency-IDD relationship indicates that there are six policy options available to prevent and control IDD:

1 Universal salt iodization.

2 Voluntary salt iodization.

3 Iodine supplementation.

4 Public health, social and agricultural development measures.

5 Nutrition education.

6 Maintaining the status quo.

Each of these policy options is described and examined in terms of how they relate to the cause of the policy problem. IDD is a policy problem resulting from inadequate iodine intake across the population and primarily caused by the existence of iodine-depleted soils. The case for each policy option as a solution to iodine deficiency disorders is assessed in relation to its public health benefits (effectiveness, cost-effectiveness, equity, and practical advantages), risks (primary and secondary and practical disadvantages), and ethical considerations, in terms of its adherence to five justificatory conditions effectiveness, proportionality, necessity, least infringement, public justification. Table 5.1 summarizes the public health benefits, risks, and ethical considerations of the six policy options available to respond to the epidemiological evidence for the iodine deficiency–IDD relationship.

The policy options are context-dependent. In other words, the assessment of each policy option will vary depending on the local circumstances associated with IDD, including:

◆ The national IDD prevalence.

◆ The level of political commitment and resources invested in the implementation of the policy option.

◆ Whether other policy interventions will be introduced to complement a particular policy option.

Therefore, the assessment of each policy option is based on three assumptions. First that IDD is prevalent in the local setting where the assessment is based; second that the level of political commitment and resources invested in each policy option is comparable with the current norms as reported in the scientific literature, i.e. not necessarily the ideal (this assumption is necessary because evidence is only available for current norms); and third, that each policy option would be implemented as a stand-alone policy response.

Universal salt iodization

Description

USI is the iodization of all salt used for human and animal consumption. Guidelines prepared by the WHO, the United Nations Children's Fund (UNICEF), and the International Council for the Control of Iodine Deficiency Disorders (ICCIDD) (14) recommend that salt be fortified with iodine at 20–40 mg iodine/kg salt, though the level of iodine fortification needs to be adjusted by national authorities in light of their own data on salt consumption patterns and the median level of urinary iodine of the population.

There are alternatives to salt as the food vehicle for delivering iodine. These alternatives include: sugar (Sudan), fish sauce (South-East Asia), animal fodder (Finland), bread—indirectly through the use of iodized baker's salt (Australia, Netherlands, and New Zealand), water (though it is a challenge to control sources and iodine has limited stability in water), oil, and milk as a side effect of iodophores used by the dairy industry (Europe, USA) (25).

However, iodine fortification of salt is widely regarded as the most effective policy intervention. This is because it is ubiquitous throughout the food supply and so is consumed by most of the population and its intake is spread evenly throughout the year. Also, iodization technology is simple and does not affect the taste or colour of salt. Its implementation is relatively inexpensive, especially as in many countries salt production and/or importation is managed by a few large companies and the quantity can be monitored at production, retail, and household level (35).

Relationship of this policy option to the cause of the policy problem

USI is a policy option that relates closely to the cause of the policy problem and the scope of the inadequate iodine intake. Adding iodine to salt compensates for the inadequate amount of this nutrient in the food supply and increases iodine exposure across the population.

Public health benefits

Effectiveness Globally, iodized salt is the most important source of dietary iodine. Its introduction has resulted in a significant reduction in the prevalence of iodine deficiency followed by a substantial decrease in the prevalence of IDD (36). In the first decade of the 21st century the prevalence of iodine deficient countries is reported to have halved (24). As the number of countries adopting USI increased substantially during the 2000s, the global prevalence in SAC of low iodine intakes fell from 36.5% (285 million) in 2003 to 29.8% (241 million) in 2011. Large decreases in prevalence during this time period occurred in Europe, the Eastern Mediterranean, South-East Asia, and the Western Pacific. However, there has been a slight increase in prevalence reported in the Americas since 2003 and little progress in Africa (28).

Cost-effectiveness USI has been reported to be the most cost-effective way of delivering iodine and of improving cognition in populations who are iodine deficient. Worldwide, the annual costs of salt iodization has been estimated at US$0.02–0.05 per child covered, with the costs per child death averted US$1000 and per disease adjusted life year gained US$34–36 (37). This conclusion is due to the relatively low cost in implementing USI, the high potential cost saving in preventing IDD, and the relatively minor public health risks and ethical considerations (see later in this assessment) associated with USI.

The economic benefit of USI was ranked especially high at Copenhagen consensus 2008. The Copenhagen consensus exercise was established to set priorities among a series of proposals for confronting ten global challenges (38). These challenges being: air pollution, conflicts, diseases, education, global warming, malnutrition and hunger, sanitation and water, subsidies and trade barriers, terrorism, and women and development. A panel of economic experts was asked to address the ten challenge areas and to answer the question: 'What would be the best ways of advancing global welfare, and particularly the welfare of the developing countries, illustrated by supposing that an additional US$75 billion of resources were at their disposal over a four-year initial period?'. Thirty options were examined across the ten challenges, micronutrient supplementation (vitamin A and zinc), micronutrient fortification (iron and salt iodization) and nutrition education were ranked as first, third, and ninth, respectively. Although this panel's findings are just one source of evidence, they have attracted much attention and as will be discussed later in this chapter they have been used by certain actors as a central plank in their advocacy activities for USI and food fortification in general.

Equity For the majority of populations, USI is an equitable intervention. It has a minimal impost on the price of food and it does not require a change in dietary behaviours, which are notoriously difficult to achieve in lower socio-economic status population groups, nor does it require individual compliance. However, there remains approximately 30% of the world's population that is not exposed to USI. This reflects various challenges with USI and in particular, its limitations in reaching those populations that are not able to access centralized food processing and distribution systems such as people living in remote areas who rely on smaller local salt producers.

Practical advantages There is no need for dietary behaviour change or ongoing compliance with special interventions because USI passively increases the public's background exposure to iodine.

Public health risks

Primary risk Excessive iodine intake that can precipitate hyperthyroidism and/or thyroiditis is the primary risk associated with USI. From 2003 to 2011 the number of countries with excessive iodine intake (median UIC >300 mg/L) increased from five to 11 (28). Excessive iodine intake is the result of poorly controlled implementation activities, e.g. during the early phase of a USI programme when salt might inadvertently be excessively iodized. A relationship between high iodine levels in drinking water and goitre prevalence has also been reported (39, 40). In addition, excessive iodine intake can result from uncoordinated intervention activities, e.g. inappropriately combining iodine supplementation programmes with USI. Uncoordinated activities are especially problematic in areas where there is adequate or even high iodine levels in drinking water and/or soils and poorly regulated or illegal distribution across national boundaries. Adverse effects of poor implementation practices can be avoided by quality assurance, monitoring, and better coordination of different intervention programmes.

Secondary risk Dietary imbalances can result from the use of salt as the delivery vehicle. Salt is a risk factor for hypertension and cardiovascular disease and dietary salt reduction can reduce cardiovascular disease risk in populations (41). In this context, there is a potential conflict between USI as a public health policy to prevent IDD using salt as the vehicle for mandatory iodine fortification and public health policies that aim to prevent cardiovascular disease by reducing salt consumption and the salt content of processed foods. Certainly there is the potential to create public confusion in relation to whether salt should be viewed as a dietary benefit or risk. However, WHO have commented that the two different public health policy agendas can be compatible (35). The recommendation that salt be fortified with iodine at a level of 20–40 mg/kg is based on the assumption of an average salt intake of approximately 5–10 g/day in adult populations, should health authorities be successful with their salt reduction campaigns and the population's salt consumption decreases the level of iodine that needs to be added to salt can be adjusted accordingly. The critical consideration in achieving a reduction in dietary salt consumption while delivering sufficient dietary iodine will be to put in place necessary coordinating mechanisms between the two distinct public health policy programmes (42).

Ethical considerations

Effectiveness USI is highly effective in preventing IDD in populations and high risk groups.

Proportionality USI is a proportional policy response in those countries where IDD is prevalent. IDD is severe and although there is a risk of excessive iodine intake which can precipitate hyperthyroidism and/or thyroiditis though usually these disorders are mild and with careful management can be transient. There is a secondary risk of compromising salt reduction programs, but the conflict can be averted if coordination is arranged between the two public health programmes.

Necessity Alternative policy options are available to help prevent IDD. However, the WHO and national authorities consistently recommend that USI is the preferred policy option.

Least infringement USI is the most coercive of the policy options available to prevent IDD. It has a high degree of infringement on an individual's free choice, especially as salt has a ubiquitous presence in the food supply and there is no immediately available dietary alternative.

Public justification The degree to which people are made aware of the impact of USI on their nutrient intake and have the opportunity to have the policy explained will vary among countries and with a range of circumstances. In many countries iodized salt is required to be labelled as such to inform citizens.

Voluntary salt iodization

Description

Voluntary salt iodization arises when decisions about if and when salt iodization might take place, what vehicle is to be used, and at what level of iodization, are determined by food manufactures and the salt industry. Voluntary salt iodization has been the common policy option implemented in HICs. Generally, under this policy option, table salt for household use is iodized, but salt used in food manufacturing tends to remain non-iodized.

Relationship of this policy option to the cause of the policy problem

Voluntary salt iodization is a policy option that relates closely to the cause of the policy problem. Adding iodine to salt on a voluntary basis helps compensate for the inadequate amount of this nutrient in the food supply and increases iodine exposure across the population. However, its coverage is variable and it may not adequately reach high risk groups within the population.

Public health benefits

Voluntary salt iodization was effective in HICs when the public chose to use iodized salt as was the norm in the middle of last century. However, in recent years as more people have reduced their discretionary addition of salt, especially in response to public health messages, and a higher proportion of salt in a non-iodized form is being derived from processed foods, iodine intake is being reduced. This is a concern because WHO prevalence data emphasize that iodine deficiency is not only a problem in LMICs. Globally, the highest prevalence of iodine deficiency occurs is in Europe where household coverage with iodized salt is low, and many European countries have weak or non-existent policies to address iodine deficiency (34). In some regions in Eastern and Western Europe where voluntary salt iodization is the common policy option, iodine deficiency that had been eliminated as a public health problem is re-emerging in a subclinical form (25). This situation has caused some to express surprise that while Western Europe has donated substantial funds towards controlling iodine deficiency in LMICs in Africa and Asia, it has not corrected its own problem (20). Those countries where voluntary salt iodization has been effective are those where there has been significant uptake of the voluntary provisions by industry, e.g. the success of Switzerland's iodized salt programme is attributed to approximately 60% of the salt used by the food industry being voluntarily iodized (20).

Voluntary salt iodization has the benefit of being a politically pragmatic policy intervention. For example, Bishai and Nalubola explain that salt iodization in the US has been voluntary particularly because the federal government does not want to be seen as interfering with individual free choice (43). They explain that the only legal incentive for US salt producers to iodize their salt relates to labelling provisions that specify iodized salt be labelled: 'This salt supplies iodide, a necessary nutrient' and uniodized salt be labelled: 'This salt does not supply iodide, a necessary nutrient' (44). Both salts are sold at the same retail price. Even though salt iodization is voluntary in the US and it is not used extensively in processed foods, it has been an effective intervention with the US enjoying among the lowest prevalence of IDD in the world. Explanations for this effectiveness include that in the US over 90% of households use iodized salt and that a relatively higher concentration of potassium iodide is used in salt in the US (20).

Public health risks

Relative to USI there is a low risk of excessive iodine intake as there is less iodized salt present in the food supply. A possible conflict with the health message to reduce salt consumption exists.

Ethical considerations

Voluntary salt iodization is proportional, though not necessary if other options are available, it is less effective than USI but at the same time it is less coercive than that policy option.

Iodine supplementation

Description

Iodine supplementation can be delivered in the form of potassium iodide or potassium iodate tablets or drops, or as iodine-vitamin complexes from the start of gestation or earlier in the case of a planned pregnancy. Iodized oil supplements are also available and can be given orally or by intramuscular injection.

Relationship of this policy option to the cause of the policy problem

Iodine supplementation relates indirectly to the cause of the policy problem. Requiring individuals to consume iodine supplements may compensate for the inadequate amount of this nutrient in the food supply but its scope is limited to increasing the iodine exposure of those individuals who regularly consume the supplements.

Public health benefits

Iodine supplementation is highly recommended by the WHO for pregnant women and young children living in high-risk communities that are unlikely to have access to iodized salt (45). It is also recommended by the WHA as a temporary strategy when salt iodization is not successfully implemented (46)—it is most frequently used in HICs. More broadly, iodine supplements may have a role in complementing 'natural' dietary sources in the circumstance where a pregnant woman might live in an iodine-sufficient area but still have a suboptimal iodine status. In this circumstance supplementation needs to be complemented with nutrition education and requires a sustained effort.

The effectiveness of iodine supplementation as a policy option has been questioned as supplements generally do not contain sufficient iodine. Pre-natal iodine supplementation in iodine-deficient regions has been shown to be associated with a significant reduction in the prevalence of endemic cretinism and infant mortality and improves cognitive function in the population (47, 48). Limited relevant evidence available to assess cost-effectiveness.

Public health risks

Public health risks in the form of acute iodine poisoning can occur as a result of excessive supplementation consumption (dose/frequency) requires behaviour change and ongoing compliance (24).

Ethical considerations

Effectiveness Supplementation can be effective when implemented as a targeted policy option for high-risk groups such as pregnant women, but as a population approach it requires wide-scale behaviour change and strict compliance.

Proportionality As a targeted public health policy intervention, supplementation is a proportional policy option as the benefits it provides to high risk groups such as pregnant women and young children outweigh the small potential risks.

Necessity Supplementation is necessary in those circumstances where USI is not being adequately implemented, but not as the primary policy option.

Least infringement Supplementation is a low coercive policy option as individuals can choose whether or not to consume supplements.

Public justification Supplementation needs to be complemented with public education approaches to promote compliance and to inform targeted individuals about potential benefits and risks.

Public health, social, and agricultural development measures

Description

Public health, social, and agricultural development measures together are used as a description for a range of policy interventions whose purpose is to promote public health conditions, alleviate poverty, and reform agricultural system. These measure are used primarily in LMICs.

Relationship of this policy option to the cause of the policy problem

Public health, social, and agricultural development measures do not relate to the cause of the policy problem, though as population-wide interventions they are consistent with the scope of inadequate iodine intake. IDD can result from iodine deficiency caused by public health problems, poverty, and 'broken' agricultural systems. In this orientation, public health, social, and agricultural development measures do relate directly to the cause and scope of the policy problem. However these circumstances are not the primary cause of IDD and not the focus of this case study.

Public health benefits

Public health, social, and agricultural development measures have many benefits associated with promoting healthy behaviours, alleviating poverty, and reforming agricultural systems. Although there is a lack of evaluative evidence available, it is anticipated that they have limited effectiveness in controlling IDD as they cannot compensate for iodine-depleted soils. Also, in many HICs the circumstances that these measures aim to address are less acute than in LMICs, despite such countries being among the most likely to experience iodine deficiency.

Public health risks

There are no apparent public health risks.

Ethical considerations

Public health, social, and agricultural development measures are a proportional policy option in the sense that there are no substantive risks to negate the potential health, social, and economic benefits that they can deliver. They have minimal infringement and are publicly justified through their focus on community development. However, they are unlikely to be effective as a stand-alone policy option, instead they provide a complement to alternative policy options.

Nutrition education

Description

Nutrition education refers to the provision of programmes and materials designed to raise the public's awareness and their skills in selecting, preparing, and consuming a healthy diet containing iodine-rich foods as far as possible within the constraints of an iodine-deficient food supply.

Relationship of this policy option to the cause of the policy problem

Nutrition education does not relate to the cause of the policy problem.

Public health benefits

There is a lack of evaluative evidence of nutrition education interventions to address IDD. Logically it would be expected that nutrition education would have limited effectiveness because it cannot compensate for iodine-depleted soils. It has the secondary benefit of raising the public's awareness and knowledge about iodine deficiency and IDD. From this perspective it is a complementary option to alternative policy interventions.

Public health risks

There are no apparent public health risks.

Ethical considerations

Nutrition education is a proportional policy option in the sense that there are no substantive risks to negate the potential benefit that arises from informing the public of the policy problem. It has minimal infringement and it is publicly justified through its explicit action in informing the public. It is unlikely to be effective as a stand-alone policy option. However, it is necessary to inform the population about the policy problem and as a complement to alternative policy options to promote a healthy balanced diet.

Maintaining the status quo

Description

Maintaining the status quo refers to deliberately deciding to not respond to epidemiological evidence of the iodine deficiency-IDD relationship. This policy option may be chosen to allow the policy maker more time to obtain additional evidence to inform an alternative policy response.

Relationship of this policy option to the cause of the policy problem

No relationship to the cause of the policy problem.

Public health benefits

There are no public health benefits of not responding to evidence of IDD resulting from population-wide iodine deficiency because there will be no increase in iodine availability in the food supply to prevent IDD.

Public health risks

There are no public health risks associated with a decision to maintain the status quo as there is no policy intervention.

When maintaining the status quo is the result of deciding to not maintain a policy option that previously had been implemented IDD may re-emerge.

Ethical considerations

Maintaining the status quo is the policy option which infringes the least on individuals and the population but it fails to meet the other four 'justificatory conditions' to support the case for this policy option: it is not effective, proportional, necessary, or publicly justified. Given the convincing evidence of the effectiveness of raised iodine exposure in controlling IDD, this policy option represents a negligent approach in those countries where there is evidence that IDD is prevalent.

Table 5.1 Summary of public health benefits, risks, and ethical considerations of policy options available to respond to the epidemiological evidence for iodine deficiency disorders

Policy option	Public health benefit	Public health risk	Ethical considerations
Universal salt iodization	High effectiveness High cost-effectiveness Equitable Does not require behaviour change Salt widely consumed and so reaches a large proportion of the population	Low–moderate risk of excessive consumption and subsequent hyperthyroidism (depending on quality control) and thyroiditis Risk of salt consumption confusing the message to reduce	High benefit for population and high-risk groups Proportional as IDD is severe and prevalent Necessary as recognised as preferred option by leading authorities Highly coercive and imposes on an individual's free choice Publicly justified, though varies across countries
Voluntary salt iodization	Moderate effectiveness though diminishes as greater proportion of salt is derived in a non-iodized form from processed foods Politically pragmatic	Low risk of excessive consumption and subsequent hyperthyroidism and thyroiditis Risk of confusing the message to reduce salt consumption	As for universal salt iodization though less effective and less coercive
Iodine supplementation	Effective for targeting high-risk groups, e.g. pregnant women Effectiveness as a population-wide intervention is dependent on behaviour change and ongoing compliance	Acute iodine poisoning if excessive supplement consumption	Low benefit for population, high benefit for high-risk groups Proportional for high risk groups, but not populations Necessary in the absence of USI Maintains individuals' free choice Publicly justified when complemented with nutrition education

Public health, social, and agricultural development measures	Lack of evidence of effectiveness in controlling IDD Secondary benefits in promoting health, social, and economic outcomes	Nil	Low benefit for population and high-risk groups proportional Moderately necessary as a complementary intervention Maintains individuals' free choice Publicly justified
Nutrition education	Lack of evidence of effectiveness in controlling IDD Secondary benefits in promoting a healthy diet Complementary intervention	Nil	Low benefit for population and high-risk groups proportional Necessary (informs the population about the policy problem and complements other policy options) Maintains individuals' free choice Publicly justified
Maintaining the status quo	Nil	IDD may re-emerge if previously controlled	No benefit for population and high-risk groups Not proportional (negligent if failing to act in those countries where there is evidence that IDD is prevalent) Not necessary Maintains individuals' free choice Not publicly justified

Analysing the policy process: chronology of the making of USI policy

A chronology of key milestones in the making of USI as a policy solution to help prevent IDD is outlined as follows.

1917–1980

In 1917, Marine and Kimball reported that goitre is caused by iodine deficiency and can be prevented with iodine supplementation (49). At this time there were no widespread food fortification precedents. Initially Marine and Kimball proposed the administration of iodine to patients directly rather than via the food supply. However, in Switzerland salt iodization as a public health policy commenced in the early 1920s as the world's first large-scale food fortification intervention (16). Closely following this Swiss initiative, several US medical professionals persuaded the Michigan State Medical Society to launch a state-wide distribution policy. The policy was implemented as a form of early

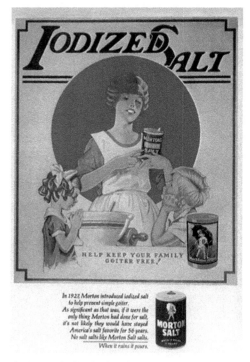

Fig. 5.2 Morton salt vintage iodized salt advert.
Reprinted with permission from Morton Salt, Inc.

public–private partnership (PPP) involving public health and medical associations working with the salt industry (43). It took some time for iodized salt to be accepted in the US more broadly. For many years the US Department of Agriculture's Bureau of Chemistry required every container of iodized salt to be marked with skull and cross-bones as iodine was considered a poison (19). These early policy developments were built upon over the next decade with salt iodization spreading to Canada, Germany, Italy, the Netherlands, New Zealand, Poland, and eventually Central and South America (19). In the 1940s, high regional goitre rates in adults and children led to recommendations by the UK's Medical Research Council for a programme of iodized salt throughout the UK (50) but no action was taken.

In 1960, WHO presented the first comprehensive international review of goitre. In spite of the review highlighting the severity and prevalence of the problem and evidence from HICs that iodized salt could successfully eliminate goitre, there was little progress made in LMICs over the next 14 years. Then in 1974 the World Food Council was the first of many international organizations that began calling for the elimination of goitre.

1980s

In the early 1980s, Hetzel proposed that the term IDDs be introduced strategically to replace the term 'goitre' because he believed it would attract greater policy interest as it drew attention to the effects of iodine deficiency on brain function (47). He was influential in championing the establishment of the ICCIDD, which was supported by WHO, UNICEF, and the Australian Government for the purpose of bridging the gap between knowledge of the policy problem and application to policy and practice (51). Then in 1986, the 39th WHA issued a resolution sponsored by Australia calling for the prevention and control of IDD. The resolution did not recommend a particular policy option; instead it urged member states to pursue: 'appropriate nutritional programmes as part of primary health care' (52).

By the late 1980s, besides Switzerland, only Australia, Canada, some of the Scandinavian countries, and the US were completely iodine sufficient. However in many other countries policy-makers were slow to recognize IDD as a major public health problem. It is during this period that the UN Sub-Committee on Nutrition established an IDD working group to receive annual report of progress on the prevention and control of IDD.

1990s

The early 1990s saw the start of concerted global action to eradicate IDD. UNICEF, WHO, and the ICCIDD were all advocating for a multi-sectoral

approach that involved national and international coalitions to blend the public-
and private-sector interests in tackling IDD. Member States at the 43rd WHA in
May 1990 agreed that WHO should aim to eliminate IDD as a public health
problem (53). Within six months, political commitment to the issue was made at
the UN world summit for children in September 1990. There 71 heads of state
and representatives of 15 governments adopted a plan of action that pledged the
virtual elimination of iodine deficiency by the year 2000 (54). In 1991, a policy
conference in Montreal, Canada: 'Ending Hidden Hunger', focusing on micronutrient malnutrition and hidden hunger, translated the political goal into policy
guidelines. A year later, the 45th WHA (7) and the WHO/Food and Agriculture
Organization international conference on nutrition agreed upon a framework of
action that would be incorporated into national nutrition strategies.

Meanwhile, studies were documenting the efficacy of daily iodized salt consumption in preventing and controlling IDD. This evidence was decisive in
influencing WHO and UNICEF (55) to adopt USI as the primary policy option
for IDD control and for it to be promoted and supported through their global
networks. Salt was chosen as the fortification vehicle because the cost of its
iodization was low, it was widely available and consumed regularly throughout
the year. UNICEF amplified its commitment through a variety of approaches
including support for national advocacy, procurement of equipment and supplies, technical assistance, and training.

In 1996 and 1999 at the 49th and 52nd WHAs, respectively, the goal to eliminate IDD as a public health problem was reaffirmed (53) in resolution
WHA49.13 (56, 57).

2000s

At the UN general assembly special session for children in 2002 a commitment
was made to achieve sustainable IDD elimination by 2005 and the Global
Network for Sustained Elimination of Iodine Deficiency was established. The
network is an alliance of ICCIDD, WHO, UNICEF, Salt Institute, EuSalt,
Kiwanis International, Micronutrient Initiative (MI), Emory University, and
the US CDC (funded from a grant of $US12 million from the Gates Foundation
through UNICEF) sharing a common commitment to assist countries to
implement USI to eliminate iodine deficiency (58).

In 2005, the 58th WHA adopted resolution 58.24 to require member states to
establish multidisciplinary national coalitions to monitor and report to the
WHA every three years on national iodine nutrition status (as indicated by
median UIC) (59). The resolution also encouraged member states to cooperate
with a range of international organizations, including UNICEF, bilateral aid
agencies, ICCIDD, MI and GAIN, to provide technical assistance to food

regulators and salt producers to support national USI implementation. Two years later, the 60th WHA (60) made special reference to applauding the support of WHO, UNICEF, World Food Programme (WFP), bilateral development agencies and nongovernmental and private partners, including Kiwanis International, ICCIDD, and the global Network for Sustained Elimination of Iodine Deficiency, for USI activities.

Progressively throughout the 2000s, PPPs were established to facilitate USI implementation. For instance, in 2008 the Bill and Melinda Gates Foundation funded a seven-year GAIN-UNICEF partnership project to reduce iodine deficiency in 13 countries with a total population of 2.3 billion: Bangladesh, China, Egypt, Ethiopia, Ghana, India, Indonesia, Niger, Pakistan, Philippines, Russia, Senegal, and Ukraine. These countries were selected based on an identified high prevalence of iodine deficiency and likelihood of successful outcomes. Several of these countries export salt to neighbouring areas and so it was expected that the scope of the project's beneficiaries would be extended (61).

2010s

In 2010 at the 63rd WHA, the progress report on: 'Sustaining the elimination of iodine deficiency disorders' highlighted the activities of the Network for Sustainable Elimination of Iodine Deficiency in supporting national efforts to eliminate IDD by promoting partnerships involving the public and private sectors and scientific and civic organizations (62).

Into the 2010s alliances are continuing to be developed to consolidate progress on IDD elimination and to achieve coverage of the remaining 30% of the world's population that is not receiving iodized salt. For example, MI and WFP have formed a partnership to support local salt processors to prepare and distribute iodized salt in six countries where iodine deficiency rates remain high: Ghana, Haiti, India, Pakistan, Sudan, and Senegal (63).

Discussion

The public health benefits, risks, and ethical considerations of universal salt iodization

USI is associated with high public health benefits in preventing and controlling IDD. Evaluative evidence consistently indicates that it is an effective intervention and the Copenhagen Consensus 2008's panel ranked it as one of the top three most cost-effective policy options for global challenges. Generally USI is equitable though it has been shown to be problematic in reaching the most vulnerable and isolated communities. It has a practical advantage in that it passively increases the iodine intake of everyone who consumes salt. USI also is associated with low-moderate public health risks. The primary risk is widespread with 11 countries in 2011 reporting excessive iodine intake among their population, though the risk can be managed with improved quality assurance practices and ongoing monitoring. A secondary risk arises from the conflicting objectives of USI and public health programmes promoting salt reduction. USI activities may require adjustments in salt iodization levels so that the aims of the salt reduction programmes can be accommodated. Ethically, USI can be justified in terms of its public health effectiveness, proportionality with benefits outweighing risks, its high level of infringement being moderated by its necessity and public justification when the community is appropriately informed and engaged with the policy.

The public health benefits, risks, and ethical considerations vary among the policy options. Relative to the five alternative policy options with which it was compared, USI is associated with higher public health benefits except for iodine supplementation which is more effective in the special case of targeting high-risk groups such as pregnant women. One qualifier in comparing the relative effectiveness of the policy options is that there is a lack of evidence that two options ('public health, social, and agricultural development measures' and 'nutrition education') have been implemented widely or evaluated for effectiveness and cost-effectiveness. None of the alternatives for which there is evidence of effectiveness available are associated with a lower public health risk than USI. Relative to USI all policy alternatives are associated with a lower infringement on an individual's free choice, but otherwise they provide a weaker ethical case based on the remaining four justificatory conditions.

There is a relationship between the degree of public health benefits, risks, and ethical considerations associated with each potential policy solution for IDD and how closely that solution matches the aetiological evidence for the underlying causation of IDD. Globally the primary underlying cause of IDD is the existence of iodine-depleted soils leading to an inherent iodine deficiency in the food supply. USI is the policy option that most directly addresses this cause. It compensates for the lack of iodine in the food supply and does so in such a way that it increases the population's iodine intake. The alternative policy options either do not directly compensate for the lack of iodine in the food supply, or if they do, their reach is not as effective as USI in delivering a population-wide coverage.

The policy process for USI

The analysis of this case study indicates that all three policy science theoretical frameworks reviewed in Chapter 2 (multiple streams, advocacy coalition framework, and network approach) have characteristics that are relevant to those observed with the USI policy-making process globally. In particular, features outlined in the network approach are supported to a significant degree by the USI policy process. For example, governments have commonly been one of many actors involved in preparing, implementing, and monitoring USI. The modern history of USI has been interwoven with a series of WHA resolutions and decisions. Initially the resolutions called for the prevention and control of IDD. In subsequent resolutions USI was specifically recommended as the preferred policy option and member states were urged to strengthen their commitments to the sustained elimination of these disorders, including regular monitoring and reporting on progress. Many member states have acted on their commitments through taking advantage of networks of interdependent relationships between actors across public and private sectors. Notably USI has been at the forefront of the global health governance arrangements (described by the network approach as an 'external factor' that influences the activities of actors within networks) that have been promoting PPPs.

The findings from this analysis have helped identify the actors involved and their relationships and activities in promoting USI. The evidence supporting USI is strong and is associated with few scientific uncertainties or ethical dilemmas. There are no major actors overtly opposing USI as a policy option to prevent and control IDD. The main actors include UN agencies (WHO, UNICEF, WFP), medical, public health, consumer, public interest non-government organizations (PINGOs), business interest non-government organizations (BINGOs), and philanthropic trusts, as well as individuals such as Professor Basil Hetzel. All have been passionate champions for USI, undertaking sustained advocacy for this policy option. For example, the Copenhagen Consensus 2008's ranking of USI as the third most cost-effective strategy to tackle global challenges produced further advocacy for increased roll-out of USI (64). The significant influence of framing activities in shaping the policy process was demonstrated with Hetzel's coining of the term IDD to replace goitre to draw attention to the seriousness of the problem and hence speed up action to achieve its elimination. Framing has also been an effective advocacy activity when the health concern has been described in graphical terms to appeal to the reader's emotions, e.g. when describing global progress on IDD prevention the president of the MI stated that this means that: 'every year, 90 million newborns' brains are protected against a significant loss of learning ability' (65).

It has been the involvement of PPPs that has been an especially critical driver of the roll-out of USI both within countries and internationally (1). These PPPs have engaged a number of UN agencies, bilateral aid agencies, philanthropic organizations, PINGOs, BINGOs, and the salt industry. The PPPs have supported the exchange of information, preparation, and distribution of iodized salt, sharing of resources, training, quality assurance, and monitoring programs, and have provided substantial financial support. It is estimated that between 1990 and 2007, nearly US$400 million in public sector investment into IDD elimination was matched by an estimated US$2 billion in salt industry investment (65). The importance placed on PPPs was the key rationale behind the establishment of the Network for Sustained Elimination of Iodine Deficiency at a special session of the UN general assembly in May 2002. The network is a PPP that brings together national governments, international organizations, the salt industry, civil society organizations, and consumer groups. Among its activities it supports the formation of 'national watches' to coordinate, harmonize, and accelerate progress on sustained iodine deficiency elimination (66).

Future directions for preventing IDD

Shortly after Marine and Kimball identified the relationship between iodine deficiency and the occurrence of goitre in 1917 (49), Marine commented: 'Simple goitre is the easiest of all known diseases to prevent... It may be excluded from the list of human diseases as soon as society determines to make the effort' (19). The technology to make this aspiration a reality exists, yet, almost 100 years later goitre has not been excluded from the list of human diseases. Certainly its prevalence has decreased substantially with the increasing adoption and implementation of USI globally. However, 32 countries are still considered iodine deficient. In Africa there has been negligible progress since 2003, with the number of school-aged children with insufficient iodine intake having increased by about 20%, from 50 to 58 million (28).

Implementing USI to reach the remaining 30% of the global population not yet covered will be a major public health policy challenge. To date, USI has been implemented in the 'easier' countries and regions in terms of their willingness and capacity to fortify and distribute iodized salt. Now it is the more economically disadvantaged communities, often living in geographically remote areas, that need to be reached. This presents logistical difficulties and added expenses with the need to work with local small-scale salt processors and rely on less reliable distribution networks. Based on critical analyses (32, 67) and a WHA resolution (46), several priority strategies are indicated for the future direction of USI. These priorities include: strengthening national coalitions to support USI, tackling uncertainties associated with measuring iodine intake and deficiency, investing in the monitoring and evaluating of programmes to control IDD (particularly for women of reproductive age and especially if pregnant or lactating), and ongoing enforcement of regulations and policy.

Lessons from the case study findings for micronutrient malnutrition and the food fortification rationale

Adding a nutrient(s) to food to compensate for the food supply being unable to provide sufficient nutrients for health was proposed as one of three plausible public health rationales for mandatory food fortification (Chapter 1, Table 1.1). Micronutrient malnutrition is the policy problem associated with this particular rationale. USI to help prevent IDD was selected as the case study for using mandatory food fortification as a policy solution for micronutrient malnutrition. In this section the findings from the assessment and analysis of the case study are generalized to identify lessons regarding the prevention of all forms of micronutrient malnutrition and the plausibility of this particular food fortification rationale. There are three particular lessons for the rationale that emerge from the generalization of this case study.

Matching a potential policy solution to the underlying cause of a policy problem

A major lesson from the assessment of this case study was the importance of matching a potential policy solution to the underlying cause of a policy problem. The degree of alignment of each policy option with the underlying cause of IDD was positively associated with the option's public health benefit, lower public health risk, and level of ethical justification. This lesson was clearly demonstrated by the positive assessment findings for USI which was the policy option most directly responding to the aetiological evidence for IDD.

There are many causes of micronutrient malnutrition among populations around the world and particularly in LMICs. USI is a representative case study of food fortification as a policy option for micronutrient malnutrition when this problem is caused by an inherent nutrient deficiency in the food supply. These findings would be expected to be generalized to other cases of micronutrient malnutrition where the cause is an inherent nutrient deficiency in the food supply. For example, the voluntary addition of niacin to cereal grain products restoring losses through grain milling and helping prevent pellagra in the US (68), although pellagra prevalence was probably declining before this fortification intervention was introduced as social circumstances and diets improved (69). Technically this case of niacin addition would be classified as restoration rather than fortification according to the Codex principles. There is less certainty about demonstrating the positive findings for the role of mandatory food fortification as a policy option for a health concern resulting from micro-nutrient malnutrition when the cause of that health concern is not related to an inherent deficiency in the food supply. For example, poverty and the lack of resources to access adequate food is a major cause of micronutrient malnutrition. In these circumstances a policy option such as a poverty alleviation programme, that directly tackles poverty and food insecurity is indicated. It would be predicted that this policy option would be associated with more public health benefits, less risks and more ethical justification than mandatory food fortification.

Predominantly, the causes of micronutrient malnutrition are embedded in a diversity of social, economic, environmental, and political circumstances that adversely affect food security in terms of reducing the availability, accessibility, and affordability of food. Indeed, in certain circumstances the primary cause of inadequate iodine intake is less due to an inherent nutrient deficiency in the food supply and more a consequence of endemic poverty. In these circumstances the public health benefits, risks, and ethical justification for food fortification as a technological option for micronutrient malnutrition need to be kept in perspective. For example, fortified foods would be expected to be efficacious in terms of increasing the availability of a nutrient(s) in a population's food supply, but often they fail to reach the poorest communities in the general population who are at the greatest risk of micronutrient deficiency. This is because such communities often have restricted access to fortified foods due to low purchasing power and an underdeveloped distribution channel. Many undernourished population groups often live on the margins of the market economy, relying on locally produced food. It is for this reason that the International Red Cross has stressed that in identifying and implementing policy options to address hunger and malnutrition there is an urgent need to tackle the underlying cause of the problem:

> The problems of chronic hunger and malnutrition are deep-seated and not amenable to quick technological fixes. They are built into the very structure of today's global food system and their solution requires political, economic, legal and social innovation and systemic changes if we are to create a well-fed world for all (70).

Into the future it is predicted that food systems are going to be placed under increasing stress in achieving food security targets in the context of an increasing global population, climate change, peak oil, and tensions over water and land use allocations. As demand for food increases and supply comes under threat, further food price rises would be expected, exacerbating social, economic, and political circumstances in which micronutrient malnutrition flourishes. Faced with this scenario there is more reason to keep food fortification as a policy solution for micronutrient malnutrition in perspective.

Some argue there is a need for policy-makers to prioritize policy options that focus less on technological fixes and more on agriculture and in particular types of food production that are more environmentally sustainable and socially just. For example, in March 2011, the UN Human Rights Council was presented with a report entitled: *Agro-ecology and the right to food* (71). The report calls on states to undertake a fundamental shift towards agroecology (the convergence of agronomy and ecology) as a mode of agricultural development for countries to feed themselves while also contributing to reducing rural poverty, improving nutrition, adapting to climate change, and promoting farmer participation in the local food system.

The SUN initiative will play a significant role in setting the global agenda for policy options, including food fortification, for micronutrient malnutrition into the future. It represents a well-resourced, broadly supported, and exciting opportunity to tackle micronutrient malnutrition. Its consensus document 'Scaling Up Nutrition' (72) has laid out a framework for action to address malnutrition focusing on encouraging governments to adopt national plans to scale up nutrition and establishing PPPs to support the implementation of these national plans.

There are two contrasting views among actors concerning the priority that food fortification should be afforded within the policy agendas for SUN. One view is that nutrient supplementation and food fortification should be priority policy options for tackling micronutrient malnutrition. This view is promoted in the report entitled *Investing in the future: a united call to action on vitamin and mineral deficiencies*. This report which was prepared by the MI, in partnership with the Flour Fortification Initiative, US Agency for International Development, Global Alliance for Improved Nutrition, WHO, The World Bank, and UNICEF, with support from the Canadian International Development Agency, promotes the view that: 'micronutrients are the best low-cost solution to improved health in the developing world' (64). An alternative view is the human rights approach captured in the report of Olivier De Schutter, the special rapporteur on the rights for food for the UN General Assembly (73) and submitted to the UN General Assembly Human Rights Council in 2011. The report identifies that food fortification has a role in circumstances where local food systems are not adequate, though generally this policy option is regarded as a short-term approach. Instead the report urges the SUN Transition Team and stakeholders to prioritize those policy options that strengthen local food systems and support the switch to sustainable diets. This view is supported by the review of Fanzo et al. who conclude that progress towards MDGs is less about developing new technologies and more about multi-sectoral programming to address poverty, gender equality, and functioning food and health systems (74).

The role of public–private partnerships

The contribution of PPP governance arrangements has been significant in facilitating the roll-out of USI and progressing the IDD elimination agenda. However, the role of PPPs in supporting food fortification in the context of micronutrient malnutrition caused by social, economic, environmental, and political circumstances is less clear cut. It would be logical to expect that partners from the private sector would be especially interested in market-based options, including the opportunity to sell fortified foods and fortificants, for micronutrient malnutrition. Transnational food and beverage manufacturers have claimed that they can be part of the micronutrient malnutrition solution by marketing various fortified snack foods and beverages in LMICs (75). Certain academics have agreed with this claim commenting that with their wide reach fortified soft drinks provide an attractive vehicle to deliver nutrients to communities in LMICs (76). Other academics argue that this approach risks promoting dietary imbalances and obesity concerns in such countries contributing to the rising prevalence of the 'double burden of malnutrition'. They also argue that the introduction of such foods and beverages will disrupt local food systems and culinary traditions (77, 78).

Plausibility of the food fortification rationale

The USI case study findings provide support for the food fortification rationale that nutrients be added to foods when the food supply is unable to provide sufficient nutrients. However, the analysis of micronutrient malnutrition problems more broadly highlights that food fortification is best implemented as a complementary intervention to public health, social, and agricultural development measures that more directly address the problems' underlying causes. The challenge in seeking such a comprehensive policy response is to ensure that a complementary relationship is achieved without one particular intervention dominating and displacing others. For example The World Bank has identified that tensions can exist between policy choices that are likely to produce a quick result, such as food fortification, but are less sustainable versus longer term, but more sustainable approaches, in tackling micronutrient malnutrition (79). The World Bank recommends the need to be strategic with food fortification, using it as a policy option in the short term to get actions underway and argues that it buys time to then move onto more sustainable, large-scale, community-based policy interventions. But does this happen in practice? The report cautions that it is important that, in using it in this way, that fortification does not take over all interventions. It urges awareness that food fortification policies do not 'crowd out attention' to more far-reaching and sustainable policy options, as has been the case in some countries in the past.

Conclusion

USI is a classic case study of using mandatory food fortification to increase a population's intake of a nutrient to help control a micronutrient malnutrition problem. It is a policy option that is technically consistent with the aetiological evidence of the underlying cause of the inadequate nutrient intake and the subsequent epidemiological evidence of the policy problem. Specifically, it is compensating for iodine-depleted soils that lead to a diminished amount of this nutrient in the food supply and iodine deficiency resulting in a high IDD prevalence. Evaluative evidence indicates that USI has been effective in preventing IDD and is associated with low-moderate risks. When these risks arise mostly they are in response to poor implementation of the policy intervention rather than an inherent problem with USI. Ethically USI is well justified and represents an intervention consistent with the utilitarian approach of striving to do the greatest good for the greatest number. Alternative policy options with which it was compared were assessed less favourably, though nutrition education and iodine supplementation are indicated as complementary interventions to strengthen USI effectiveness.

Many actors are involved with USI. They have formed powerful advocacy coalitions to not just place IDD problems onto the political agenda but to continually advocate for maintaining USI as a global public health policy priority. They have framed the policy problem directly around the substantial amount of evidence that is available, evidence that is convincing and associated with few uncertainties. Globally, the development of USI and its roll-out across the majority of countries has been facilitated by powerful and particularly active PPPs. These PPPs have engaged a number of UN agencies, philanthropic organizations, PINGOs, and BINGOs.

Generalizing the findings from this case study to food fortification as a policy solution for micronutrient malnutrition overall and to assess the plausibility of the food fortification rationale provides valuable lessons. There are multiple causes of micronutrient malnutrition. Evidence from other studies indicates that when the cause of micronutrient malnutrition relates to social, economic, or political circumstances, rather than an inherent nutrient deficiency in the food supply, the case for food fortification as a policy option needs to be kept in perspective. Depending on the underlying cause and the particular circumstances associated with micronutrient malnutrition, food fortification may play a complementary role to other policy options in compensating for the food supply being unable to provide a sufficient amount of a nutrient(s).

References

1. World Health Organization. *Micronutrient deficiencies. Iodine deficiency disorders.* [cited 12 April 2012]. Available from: http://www.who.int/nutrition/topics/idd/en/.

2. World Health Organization. *Micronutrient deficiencies. Vitamin A deficiency.* [cited 25 September 2012]. Available from: www.who.int/nutrition/topics/vad/en/.

3. World Health Organization. *Micronutrient deficiencies. Iron deficiency anaemia.* [cited 25 September 2012]. Available from: www.who.int/nutrition/topics/ida/en/index.html.

4. Black R. Micronutrient deficiency—an underlying cause of morbidity and mortality. *Bulletin of the World Health Organization* 2008; 81(2):79.

5. Caulfield LE, Black RE. Zinc deficiency. *Comparative quantification of health risks: global and regional burden of disease attributable to selected major risk factors.* Geneva: WHO; 2004.

6. Darnton-Hill I, Webb P, Harvey PW, Hunt JM, Dalmiya N, Chopra M, *et al.* Micronutrient deficiencies and gender: social and economic costs. *American Journal of Clinical Nutrition* 2005; 81(5):1198S–205S.

7. World Health Organization. *WHA45.33 National strategies for prevention and control of micronutrient malnutrition, Geneva, 4–14 May.* Geneva: WHO; 1992 [cited 11 August 2011]. Available from: http://www.who.int/nutrition/topics/wha_nutrition_mnm/en/index.html.

8. United Nations System Standing Committee on Nutrition. *Sixth report on the world nutrition situation.* Geneva: UNSCN; 2010 [cited 26 February 2012]. Available from: http://www.unscn.org/files/Publications/RWNS6/html/index.html.

9. World Health Organization. *Recommendations on wheat and maize flour fortification meeting report: interim consensus statement.* 2009 [cited 28 March 2012]. Available from: http://www.who.int/nutrition/publications/micronutrients/wheat_maize_fortification/en/index.html.

10. United Nations International Children's Emergency Fund. [cited 23 January 2012]. Available from: http://www.unicef.org/media/media_23416.html.

11. Darnton-Hill I, Nalubola R. Fortification strategies to meet micronutrient needs: successes and failures. *Proceedings of The Nutrition Society* 2002; 61(2):231–41.

12. United Nations. *Millennium Development Goals* [cited 25 September 2012]. Available from: http://www.un.org/millenniumgoals/.

13. United Nations System Standing Committee on Nutrition. *Scaling Up Nutrition: A Framework for Action. Based on a series of consultations hosted by the Center for Global Development, the International Conference on Nutrition.* Geneva: USAID, UNICEF and the World Bank; 2010.

14. World Health Organization/United National Children's Fund/International Council for the Control of Iodine Deficiency Disorders. *Assessment of iodine deficiency disorders and monitoring their elimination. A guide for programme managers.* Geneva: World Health Organization; 2007.

15. Zimmermann MB, Jooste PL, Pandav CS. Iodine-deficiency disorders. *Lancet* 2008; 372(9645):1251–62.

16. Burgi H, Supersaxo Z, Selz B. Iodine deficiency diseases in Switzerland one hundred years after Theodor Kocher's survey: a historical review with some new goitre prevalence data. *Acta Endocrinologica (Copenhagen)* 1990; 123(6):577–90.

17. Zimmermann M. Research on iodine deficiency and goiter in the 19th and early 20th centuries. *Journal of Nutrition* 2008; 138(11):2060–3.

18. Rosenfeld L. Discovery and early uses of iodine. *Journal of Chemical Education* 2000; 77:984–7.

19. World Health Organization. *World Health Organization Monograph Series No. 44: Endemic goitre.* Geneva: WHO; 1960.

20. Zimmerman M. Iodine deficiency in industrialised countries. *Proceedings of the Nutrition Society* 2010; 69:133–43.

21. Li M, Waite KV, Ma G, Eastman CJ. Declining iodine content of milk and re-emergence of iodine deficiency in Australia. *Medical Journal of Australia* 2006; 184(6):307.

22. Institute of Medicine of the National Academies. *Dietary reference intakes for vitamin A, vitamin K, arsenic, boron, chromium, copper, iodine, iron, manganese, molybdenum, nickel, silicon, vanadium and zinc.* Washington, DC: Institute of Medicine of the National Academies; 2001.

23. WHO/PAHO Regional Expert Group for Cardiovascular Disease Prevention (ed). *Improving public health in the Americas by optimizing sodium and iodine intakes.* Washington DC: WHO/PAHO; 2011.

24. Speeckaert M, Speeckaert R, Wierckx K, Delanghe J, Kaufman J-M. Value and pitfalls in iodine fortification and supplementation in the 21st century. *British Journal of Nutrition* 2011; 106:964–73.

25. Allen L, de Benoist B, Dary O, Hurrell R. *Guidelines on food fortification with micronutrients.* Geneva: World Health Organization; 2006 [cited 25 September 2012]. Available from: http://www.who.int/nutrition/publications/guide_food_fortification_micronutrients.pdf.

26. Zimmermann MB, Jooste PL, Mabapa NS, Mbhenyane X, Schoeman S, Biebinger R, *et al.* Treatment of iodine deficiency in school-age children increases insulin-like growth factor (IGF)-I and IGF binding protein-3 concentrations and improves somatic growth. *Journal of Clinical Endocrinology and Metabolism* 2007; 92(2):437–42.

27. Zimmermann MB. Iodine deficiency in pregnancy and the effects of maternal iodine supplementation on the offspring: a review. *American Journal of Clinical Nutrition* 2009; 89(2):668S–72S.

28. Andersson M, Karumbunathan V, Zimmermann MB. Global iodine status in 2011 and trends over the past decade. *Journal of Nutrition* 2012; 142(4):744–50.

29. Als C, Haldimann M, Burgi E, Donati F, Gerber H, Zimmerli B. Swiss pilot study of individual seasonal fluctuations of urinary iodine concentration over two years: is age-dependency linked to the major source of dietary iodine? *European Journal of Clinical Nutrition* 2003; 57(5):636–46.

30. Mian C, Vitaliano P, Pozza D, Barollo S, Pitton M, Callegari G, *et al.* Iodine status in pregnancy: role of dietary habits and geographical origin. *Clinical Endocrinology (Oxford)* 2009; 70(5):776–80.

31. Moreno-Reyes R, Carpentier YA, Macours P, Gulbis B, Corvilain B, Glinoer D, *et al.* Seasons but not ethnicity influence urinary iodine concentrations in Belgian adults. *European Journal of Nutrition* 2010; 50(4):285–90.

32. Zimmermann MB. Iodine deficiency. *Endocrine Reviews* 2009; 30(4):376–408.

33. Delange F, Lecomte P. Iodine supplementation: benefits outweigh risks. *Drug Safety* 2000; 22(2):89–95.

34. World Health Organization. *Iodine deficiency in Europe: a continuing health problem.* Geneva: WHO; 2007.

35. World Health Organization. *Salt as a vehicle for fortification. Report of a WHO Expert Consultation. Luxembourg, 21–22 March 2007.* Geneva: WHO; 2008.

36. Deitchler M, Mathys E, Mason J, Winichagoon P, Tuazon MA. Lessons from successful micronutrient programs. Part II: program implementation. *Food and Nutrition Bulletin* 2004; 25(1):30–52.

37. Caulfield L, Richard, SA, Rivera, JA, Musgrove P, Black RE. Stunting, wasting, and micronutrient deficiency disorders. In: Jamison D, Breman JG, Measham AR, Alleyne G, Claeson M, Evans DB, *et al.* (eds). In: *Disease Control Priorities in Developing Countries*, 2nd ed. New York: Oxford University Press; 2006, pp. 551–68.

38. Copenhagen Consensus. Available from: http://www.copenhagenconsensus.com/ Home.aspx].

39. Shen H, Liu S, Sun D, Zhang S, Su X, Shen Y, *et al.* Geographical distribution of drinking-water with high iodine level and association between high iodine level in drinking-water and goitre: a Chinese national investigation. *British Journal of Nutrition* 2011; 15:1–5.

40. Henjum S, Barikmo I, Gjerlaug AK, Mohamed-Lehabib A, Oshaug A, Strand TA, *et al.* Endemic goitre and excessive iodine in urine and drinking water among Saharawi refugee children. *Public Health Nutrition* 2010; 13(9):1472–7.

41. Bibbins-Domingo K, Chertow GM, Coxson PG, Moran A, Lightwood JM, Pletcher MJ, *et al.* Projected effect of dietary salt reductions on future cardiovascular disease. *New England Journal of Medicine* 2010; 362(7):590–9.

42. Campbell N, Dary O, Cappuccio FP, Neufeld LM, Harding KB, Zimmermann MB. Collaboration to optimize dietary intakes of salt and iodine: a critical but overlooked public health issue. *Bulletin of the World Health Organization* 2012; 90(1):73–4.

43. Bishai D, Nalubola R. The history of food fortification in the United States: its relevance for current fortification efforts in developing countries. *Economic Development and Cultural Change* 2002; 51(1):37–53.

44. US Government. *Title 21 Code of Federal Regulations* Washington DC: US Government Printing Office; 2000.

45. World Health Organization/United Nations Children's Fund. *Joint Statement: Reaching optimal iodine nutrition in pregnant and lactating women and young children.* Geneva: WHO/UNICEF; 2007.

46. World Health Organization. *2010 WHA 63/27: Sustaining the elimination of iodine deficiency disorders (resolution WHA60.21).* [cited 26 April 2012]. Available from: http://www.who.int/nutrition/topics/A63.27_idd_en.pdf.

47. Hetzel BS. Iodine deficiency disorders (IDD) and their eradication. *Lancet* 1983; 2(8359):1126–9.

48. Pharoah PO, Connolly KJ. A controlled trial of iodinated oil for the prevention of endemic cretinism: a long-term follow-up. *International Journal of Epidemiology* 1987; 16(1):68–73.

49. Marine D, Kimball OP. The prevention of simple goitre in man. *Journal of Laboratory and Clinical Medicine* 1917; 3:40–8.

50. Medical Research Council Vitamin Study Research Group. Prevention of neural tube defects: Results of the Medical Research Council Vitamin Study. *Lancet* 1991 338:131–7.

51. Semba RD. The historical evolution of thought regarding multiple micronutrient nutrition. *Journal of Nutrition* 2012; 142(1):143S–56S.

52. World Health Assembly. *WHA39.31 Prevention and control of iodine deficiency disorders, Geneva, 5–16 May 1986.* [cited 26 April 2012]. Available from: http://www.who.int/nutrition/topics/WHA39.31_idd_en.pdf.

53. World Health Assembly. *Resolution WHA43.2 Prevention and control of iodine deficiency disorders, Geneva, 7–17 May 1990.* [cited 28 April 2012]. Available from: http://www.who.int/nutrition/topics/WHA43.2_idd_en.pdf.

54. United Nations Chidren's Fund. *First call for children. World declaration and plan of action from the World Summit for Children.* UNICEF: New York; 1990.

55. United Nations Chidren's Fund/World Health Organization. *UNICEF-WHO Joint Committee on Health Policy. World Summit for Children mid-decade goal: iodine deficiency disorders (IDD). UNICEF-WHO Joint Committee on Health Policy, Special Session, 27–28 January 1994.* Geneva: UNICEF/WHO; 1994.

56. World Health Assembly. *WHA49.13 Prevention and control of iodine deficiency disorders, Geneva, 20–25 May 1996.* [cited 28 April 2012]. Available from: http://www.who.int/nutrition/topics/WHA49.13_idd_en.pdf.

57. World Health Assembly. *WHA52.24 Prevention and control of iodine deficiency disorders, Geneva, 17–25 May 1999.* [cited 28 April 2012]. Available from: http://www.who.int/nutrition/topics/WHA52.24_idd_en.pdf.

58. International Council for the Control of Iodine Deficiency Disorders. [cited 3 June 2012]. Available from: http://www.iccidd.org/index.php.

59. World Health Assembly. *WHA58.24 Sustaining the elimination of iodine deficiency disorders, Geneva, 16–25 May 2005.* [cited 29 April 2012]. Available from: http://www.who.int/nutrition/topics/WHA58.24_idd_en.pdf.

60. World Health Assembly. *WHA60.21 Sustaining the elimination of iodine deficiency disorders, Geneva, 14–23 May 2007.* [cited 28 April 2012]. Available from: http://www.who.int/nutrition/topics/WHA60.21_idd_en.pdf.

61. Global Alliance for Improved Nutrition. [cited 25 September 2012]. Available from: http://www.gainhealth.org/programs/USI.

62. World Health Assembly. *WHA 63/27:A63/27, Progress reports—Sustaining the elimination of iodine deficiency disorders (WHA60.21), Geneva, 15 April 2010.* [cited 26 April 2012]. Available from: http://www.who.int/nutrition/topics/A63.27_idd_en.pdf.

63. Micronutrient Initiative. [cited 30 April 2012]. Available from: http://www.micronutrient.org/English/View.asp?x=578.

64. Micronutrient Initiative. *Micronutrient Initiative, Investing in the future: A united call to action on vitamin and mineral deficiencies, Global report 2009.* [cited 30 April 2012]. Available from: http://ww.unitedcalltoaction.org.

65. Mannar VMG. Eliminating iodine deficiency: Learning from an untold public health success story. [Editorial] *SCN News, Universal Salt Iodization* 2007; 35:3–4.

66. Dalmiya N, Schultink W. Combating hidden hunger: the role of international agencies. *Food and Nutrition Bulletin* 2003; 24(4 Suppl):S69–77.

67. Dunn JT. Seven deadly sins in confronting endemic iodine deficiency, and how to avoid them. *Journal of Clinical Endocrinology & Metabolism* 1996; 81(4):1332–5.

68. Park YK, Sempos CT, Barton CN, Vanderveen JE, Yetley EA. Effectiveness of food fortification in the United States: the case of pellagra. *American Journal of Public Health* 2000; 90(5):727–38.

69. Nestle M. Folate fortification and neural tube defects: policy implications. *Journal of Nutrition Education* 1994; 26(6):287–93.

70. International Federation of Red Cross and Red Crescent Societies. *World Disasters Report 2011—Focus on hunger and malnutrition. IFRC/RCS*: Geneva, Switzerland. [cited 27 September 2011]. Available from: http://redcross.org.au/files/World_Disasters_Report_FINAL.pdf.

71. United Nations Human Rights Council. *Agroecology and the Right to Food, Report presented at the 16th Session of the United Nations Human Rights Council [A/HRC/16/49], 8 March 2011.* [cited 29 September 2011]. Available from: http://www.srfood.org/index.php/en/component/content/article/1174-report-agroecology-and-the-right-to-food.

72. Bezanson K, Isenman P. Scaling up nutrition: a framework for action. *Food and Nutrition Bulletin*; 31(1):178–86.

73. United Nations General Assembly Human Rights Council. *Report submitted by the Special Rapporteur on the right to food, Oliver De Schutter. Nineteenth session. A/HRC/19/59. Agenda item 3. 26 December 2011.* Geneva: United Nations; [cited 25 September 2012]. Available from: http://www2.ohchr.org/english/bodies/hrcouncil/docs/19session/A.HRC.19.59_English.pdf.

74. Fanzo JC, Pronyk PM. A review of global progress toward the Millennium Development Goal 1 hunger target. *Food and Nutrition Bulletin* 2012; 32(2):144–58.

75. Yach D, Feldman ZA, Bradley DG, Khan M. Can the food industry help tackle the growing global burden of undernutrition? *American Journal of Public Health* 2010; 100(6):974–80.

76. Wojcicki JM, Heyman MB. Malnutrition and the role of the soft drink industry in improving child health in sub-Saharan Africa. *Pediatrics* 2010; 126(6):e1617–21.

77. Monteiro CA, Gomes FS, Cannon G. The snack attack. *American Journal of Public Health* 2010; 100(6):975–81.

78. Nestle M. *Soft drinks as a solution to childhood malnutrition? I don't think so. Marion Nestle blog, 'Food Politics' posted on 18 November 2010.* [cited 12 October 2011]. Available from: http://www.foodpolitics.com/tag/fortification/.

79. The World Bank. *Repositioning nutrition as central to development.* 2006 [cited 27 April 2012]. Available from: http://siteresources.worldbank.org/NUTRITION/Resources/281846-1131636806329/NutritionStrategy.pdf.

Chapter 6

Case study 2: mandatory flour fortification with folic acid

Adding a biologically active ingredient to the food supply of 300 million people is a very weighty issue. You can't experiment on the American people.

(Personal communication, 26 July 2012, Professor David Kessler, former Commissioner of the US Food and Drug Administration.)

Introduction

Conventionally, mandatory flour fortification with folic acid (MFFFA) has been implemented as a policy option to help prevent and control micronutrient malnutrition such as child and maternal anaemia associated with folate deficiency (1). Then, in the mid-1990s, policy-makers in some countries began considering using MFFFA under a novel policy paradigm. The paradigm operated from the view that MFFFA be used to increase the folic acid intake of certain individuals who had an increased requirement for this nutrient irrespective of the folate status of the population as a whole.

The new policy view was prompted by the need to respond to convincing epidemiological evidence that increasing the folic acid intake for certain women reduced their risk of having a neural tube defect (NTD)-affected pregnancy. NTDs are congenital malformations of the central nervous system resulting from the failure of the neural tube to close during embryogenesis and most commonly include spina bifida and anencephaly. They place a devastating health, social, financial, and emotional burden on affected individuals and their families. National NTD birth prevalence varies widely depending on genetic and environmental conditions and has been recorded as high as six per 1000 live births in China (2). Over 95% of all NTDs are first occurrence, with a small proportion being recurrent events in women with a previously affected pregnancy (3).

In this orientation MFFFA was (and remains today) a controversial policy intervention. As will be described in this chapter it is associated with many scientific uncertainties and ethical dilemmas. In responding to the epidemiological evidence policy-makers have struggled to formulate a policy that promotes the health interests of at-risk individuals while protecting the health of the wider population. As illustrated in the opening quote to this chapter, the former Commissioner of the US Food and Drug Administration (FDA) at the time that MFFFA was first being debated in the US alludes to the policy in terms that have connotations of 'medicalizing' the food supply and as such, he could not take the decision lightly. In this context the medicalization of the food supply refers to the imposition of a biomedical remit (4) onto how the relationship between food and health is viewed. By extension food is regarded as a form of therapeutic agent with the purpose of helping treat or prevent a disease.

The decision-making process for translating the evidence of the folic acid-NTD relationship into a policy response is associated with a number of scientific uncertainties, complicating factors and ethical dilemmas. It is the existence of this peculiar combination of circumstances that makes MFFFA an especially powerful food fortification case study. At the time that MFFFA was first being implemented, the editor of one international nutrition journal described the relationship of folic acid to neural tube defects as providing, 'one of the richest case studies in nutrition science policy of this half century'(5). By 2009, there were a number of countries that were contemplating whether or not to introduce MFFFA. In response, the World Health Organization (WHO) disseminated guidelines on levels of folic acid fortification for wheat and maize flour recommending fortification at 1.0 to 5.0 ppm, depending on a country's wheat flour consumption per capita (6).

The purpose of this chapter is to present the findings of the investigation into the MFFFA case study. The chapter starts by outlining the background to the case study. Then an assessment of the case study's public health benefits, risks, and ethical considerations relative to alternative policy options is presented followed by a chronology of key milestones in the making of MFFFA policy. A discussion of the assessment findings and of the analysis of the actors, activities, and agendas surrounding the chronology to help explain how and why the policy was made, is provided. Emerging from the discussion are proposed future directions for preventing NTDs. Finally the case study findings are generalised to construct lessons regarding the plausibility of the food fortification rationale that adding nutrients to food is evidence-informed and ethically justified in circumstances where certain individuals have nutrient requirements higher than reference standards.

Background

Folate and health

Folate is a water soluble B-group vitamin and the generic name for a group of structurally-related compounds that are both naturally occurring and synthetic. The natural form of folate (pterolypolyglutamate) was identified by Wills in 1931 (7). Several years later a synthetic version of the vitamin, which rarely occurs naturally in food, folic acid (pteroylmonoglutamate), was produced (8). Folic acid is more bioavailable in the human body and stable in food processing, manufacture, and storage than folate (9). Folic acid is the form of the vitamin used for supplements (either alone or in multivitamin complexes) and food fortification.

There are many critical biochemical pathways that are dependent on folate. It is a one-carbon substrate in nucleic acid and amino acid metabolism required for the synthesis of DNA and RNA, for the conversion of the amino acid homocysteine to methionine, as well as for DNA, RNA, and protein methylation (10). Due to the importance of folate in DNA and RNA synthesis, folate requirements are increased during times of rapidly dividing cellular tissue such as red blood cell formation, and for fetal development.

Food sources of folate

Folate is ubiquitous in the food supply. Particularly good food sources of folate include green leafy vegetables such as broccoli and spinach, legumes such as beans, and citrus fruits and juices (see Figure 6.1).

Recommended intake levels

The recommended daily folate intake levels for different population groups vary among countries around the world, and by age and sex (11). In the US, the folate reference dietary allowance for all males and non-pregnant females ≥14 years is 400 μg of dietary folate equivalents (the term 'dietary folate equivalents' is used to accommodate the varying bioavailabilities of folate and folic acid) and increases to 600 and 500 μg dietary folate equivalents/day for pregnant and lactating women respectively.

Folate metabolism is well regulated and as such it is regarded as safe at any level of intake. Folic acid metabolism is not as well regulated and unmetabolized folic acid has been detected in the circulatory system following mandatory (12) and voluntary (13) folic acid fortification. The public health and safety implications of the presence of novel levels of unmetabolized folic acid in the circulatory system are a source of much debate. As Smith has commented (14):

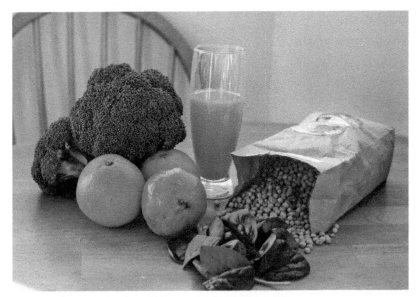

Fig. 6.1 Selected foods that are good sources of folate.

> But folate being involved in so many of life's fundamental processes not only leads to
> its possibilities as a panacea but also to the prospect that 'messing around with folate'
> could do extensive harm.

One particular concern is that a high level of folic acid intake can mask the symptoms of vitamin B12 deficiency and delay its diagnosis thus exacerbating subsequent neurological damage (15). As a consequence, the tolerable upper intake level (UL) for folic acid intake is set at 1 mg/d (16).

Given folate's central role in many biochemical pathways it is not surprising that evidence is available linking novel intakes of folic acid with a range of health outcomes throughout the lifecycle. These health outcomes include: promoting twinning during pregnancy (17), promoting atopic dermatitis in newborns (18), promoting asthma during childhood (19), and promoting (20) and protecting against (21) cognitive decline in older adults.

Folic acid's proposed dual role with regard to the risk of certain cancers (22) that has attracted particular attention from researchers and policy-makers. Increasing the folic acid intake of an individual experiencing folate deficiency may be protective against cancer. Conversely some epidemiological studies have provided evidence that an increased folic acid intake facilitates the progression of pre-neoplastic cells and promotes colorectal cancer (23–24). However, subsequent studies have concluded that there is a lack of evidence that exposure to high levels of folic acid is a risk factor for promoting the progression of colorectal cancer (25–27) and there may be an association with a decreased risk (28). Although the concern has subsided to some degree, there remains lingering doubt about the safety of increased folic acid intake in relation to risk of promoting the progression of colorectal cancer (29). With a latency period of between 10–20 years from the initial adverse exposure to the detection of colorectal cancer this remains a priority area for ongoing monitoring.

Epidemiological evidence for the policy problem

The importance of nutrition in the aetiology of NTDs was first suggested by Hibbard et al. in the mid-1960s (30). Then in the early 1990s, epidemiological evidence emerged from trials with folic acid supplements that sufficient folic acid consumed during the periconceptional period (one month pre-conception to three months post-conception) helps to reduce the risk of recurrence (31) and occurrence (32) of NTDs. A systematic review, following the Cochrane procedures, of further studies using folic acid supplementation has confirmed the protective effect of folic acid supplementation on NTDs (33). However, the optimum and indeed minimum dose of folic acid necessary to reduce the risk of NTDs is uncertain (34). Given the convincing epidemiological evidence for the relationship it would be unethical to conduct further trials deliberately denying individuals access to folic acid so as to help estimate a precise optimum and minimum dose. Related to this uncertainty, is whether or not there might be a contributing protective role from other nutrients, such as vitamin B12, that share common metabolic pathways with folic acid.

Cause of the policy problem

NTDs have an uncertain multifactorial aetiology involving a combination of genetic and environmental factors. Nutrition is the most significant environmental factor, particularly because of the protective effect of folic acid. However, not all NTD cases can be prevented by the administration of folic acid. Trials using high doses of folic acid supplements have demonstrated an approximate 70% protective effect, i.e. 30% of cases were not prevented. In countries where MFFFA has been implemented, the NTD birth prevalence is resistant to attempts to reduce the rate below five cases per 10,000 births revealing an apparent 'floor effect' for folic acid-preventable NTD (35). Other environmental factors are independent risks, e.g. maternal weight (36). In addition it is reported that NTDs exhibit a social gradient with prevalence being associated with economic disadvantage and maternal education status (37).

The protective mechanism(s) through which folic acid reduces the risk of NTDs is not known. It is known that folate requirements can be affected by genetic variants. A number of genetic polymorphisms affect folate pathways and metabolism, and have been associated with an increased risk for NTDs (38). In particular, women who are homozygous for the T allele of the C677T polymorphism of the gene encoding the folate dependent enzyme 5,10 methylene-tetrahydrofolate reductase have a raised requirement for folate and are at increased risk of experiencing an NTD-affected pregnancy (39). Moreover, observed ethnic differences in the frequency of the C677T polymorphism, ranging from 0% in African American women to 3.8%, 7.2%, and 18.1% in Asian, white and Mexican women respectively, indicate ethnic variations in folate requirements (40).

What is apparent is that folic acid exerts its protective influence by acting more as a therapeutic agent than as a conventional nutrient. The 'dose' of folic acid required to reduce the risk of NTDs is in addition to that required for an otherwise adequate folate intake; it is not therefore compensating for a conventional folate deficiency. A dose-response relationship between folic acid and NTD incidence and severity has been demonstrated (41–43).

Challenges with translating the epidemiological evidence for the policy problem into a policy solution

Governments all over the world are struggling to identify the best policy response to the convincing epidemiological evidence of the folic acid–NTD relationship. On first blush the selection of a policy option may appear a straightforward matter—promote folic acid supplements to those women who might be genetically predisposed to being at risk of having an NTD-affected pregnancy. This policy option is consistent with the nature of the folic acid supplement trials that provided the convincing evidence, the dose of folic acid in the supplement can be precisely controlled and the supplement can be delivered as a targeted 'treatment' to genetically susceptible individuals. However, there are scientific uncertainties and complicating circumstances that result in the evidence translation process being less straightforward than might otherwise be anticipated.

The primary scientific uncertainty is the unknown mechanism(s) by which folic acid reduces the risk of NTDs. This means that it is not possible to identify a genetically susceptible woman, apart from those women who have previously had an NTD-affected pregnancy where this places them at increased risk of recurrence. This situation is exacerbated by complicating circumstances such as the estimation that approximately half of all pregnancies are unplanned (44) and so many women may not be aware of the need to take a folic acid supplement in preparation for pregnancy. In addition the neural tube closes by approximately the 28th day after conception, a date at which a woman may be unaware that she is pregnant and so would not appreciate the need to take a folic acid supplement. This combination of scientific uncertainties and complicating circumstances effectively means that policy options need to be directed at a target group, 'women of child bearing age', and not specific individuals.

Assessing the public health benefits, risks, and ethical considerations of policy options

There are five policy options available to respond to the epidemiological evidence for the folic acid–NTD relationship:

1 Mandatory flour fortification with folic acid.

2 Voluntary flour fortification with folic acid.

3 Folic acid supplementation.

4 Nutrition education.

5 Maintaining the status quo.

Each of these policy options is described and examined in terms of how they relate to the cause of the policy problem. NTDs are a policy problem resulting primarily from a presumed genetic polymorphism affecting the ability of genetically susceptible individuals to efficiently metabolize folate in the diet. The case for each policy option as a solution to NTDs is assessed in relation to its public health benefits (effectiveness, cost-effectiveness, equity and practical advantages), risks (primary and secondary and practical disadvantages), and risks and ethical considerations, in terms of its adherence to five justificatory conditions effectiveness, proportionality, necessity, least infringement, public justification. Table 6.1 summarizes the public health benefits, risks and ethical considerations of the five policy options.

The policy options are context-dependent. The assessment of each policy option will vary depending on the local circumstances associated with NTDs, including:

◆ The national baseline prevalence of NTDs and folate status.

◆ The proportion of unplanned pregnancies.

◆ The level of support that is provided to implement the policy option.

◆ Whether other policy interventions will be introduced to complement a particular policy option.

◆ The national frequency of the 677 TT polymorphism

Therefore, the assessment of each policy option is based on five assumptions. First, that national NTD prevalence and folate status is moderate relative to international norms; second, that the proportion of unplanned pregnancies is approximately 50%; third, that the level of political support for each policy option is comparable with the current norms, i.e. not necessarily the ideal (this assumption is necessary because evidence is only available for current norms); fourth, that each policy option would be implemented as a stand-alone policy response; and fifth, that the national frequency of the 677 TT polymorphism is 9% (the mid-point of observed ethnic variations).

Mandatory flour fortification with folic acid

Description

MFFFA is a policy intervention in which a government regulates for the compulsory addition of folic acid to flour. As mentioned earlier, the WHO recommendations on wheat and maize flour fortification specify folic acid fortification at 1.0–5.0ppm, depending on a country's wheat flour consumption per capita (6). Wheat flour is the most widely consumed cereal grain in the world and the fortification technology with roller mills is simple and does not affect the taste or colour of flour (45).

Relationship of this policy option to the cause of the policy problem

MFFFA does not directly address the cause of the policy problem. Adding folic acid to flour increases the folic acid intake of genetically susceptible individuals (assuming they consume fortified flour products). Therefore, it helps them consume a dose of folic acid to indirectly 'compensate' for the presumed genetic defect that predisposes them to an increased risk of having an NTD-affected pregnancy.

Public health benefits

Effectiveness MFFFA has been shown to be effective in helping prevent NTDs. A meta-analysis of NTD prevention studies reports that MFFFA can reduce the incidence of NTDs by 46% (46). However, it is possible that these reported levels of effectiveness are an over-estimate because typically they do not take into account any increase in folic acid consumption contributed by supplements or voluntarily fortified foods that are usually promoted during MFFFA implementation. MFFFA effectiveness has been observed to vary with the baseline NTD prevalence and folate status of populations in different countries (35, 47). For instance in countries such as the US that enter into a MFFFA intervention with a relatively high pre-existing folic acid presence in the food supply, NTD prevalence reductions of 20–30% have been reported (48). At the other end of the effectiveness scale, in Costa Rica where there was a lower folic acid presence when MFFFA was implemented, an NTD reduction of 58% has been reported (49).

A secondary public health benefit is that in those countries with folate deficiency, MFFFA will increase folic acid intake to help prevent anaemia. Though evidence of a population-wide folate deficiency resulting in a high prevalence of anaemia might be expected to be the primary motivation for a MFFFA policy decision and NTD-prevention would be the secondary beneficiary of such a policy decision.

Cost-effectiveness Cost-effectiveness studies of MFFFA can be problematic sources of evidence to inform policy-making for this policy problem. The methods used to conduct research have varied among researchers, the findings have not always been consistent and questionable assumptions have been made in their interpretation. Studies have reported that MFFFA is a cost-effective policy option (50). One study reported that MFFFA is less cost-effective than a combination of supplementation and voluntary fortification (see below). Frequently, the evidence provided from different studies has varied depending on what benefits and risks were included in the research design and how they were measured. For example, one study included myocardial infarction prevention as a benefit of MFFFA (51) despite a lack of evidence for such an inclusion. Few studies have considered the costs associated with the ethical considerations of MFFFA. Some actors cite the positive Copenhagen Consensus (Chapter 4) cost-effectiveness findings towards micronutrient programmes to support MFFFA although that exercise was based on iron and iodine fortification and supplementation (vitamin A and zinc) was ranked as more cost-effective than fortification. Few studies have undertaken a cost-effective analysis comparing the different policy options.

Equity MFFFA increases the folic acid intake of everyone in the population who consumes folic acid-fortified flour products. It does this without the need for behaviour change and hence may equitably reach at-risk individuals in disadvantaged groups. Estimating the extent of this equity advantage relative to conventional health promotion and folic acid supplementation policy options is problematic (52). MFFFA does not significantly affect the price or taste of fortified foods. Because MFFFA is a non-targeted intervention it cannot take into account social and cultural variations among communities, e.g. after MFFFA was introduced in the US it has been observed that Hispanic populations have a 30–40% higher risk of NTDs (53) and this is linked to these populations eating less of the fortified foods than the population average.

Practical advantages The key practical advantage of MFFFA is that it removes the need for the target group to change its dietary behaviour to help achieve the recommended folic acid intake because MFFFA passively increases the target group's (and population's) background exposure to folic acid. This explains its effectiveness and equitable nature. In addition the government is responsible for implementation so it has control over the timing, levels and extent of fortification.

Public health risks

Primary risk Policy-makers face a balancing act in selecting foods to be fortified and then setting the level of fortification so that a sufficient folic acid dose is delivered to the target group, while avoiding increasing the folic acid intake of the target group and population beyond the UL for this nutrient. The risks associated with excessive folic acid intake resulting from the non-targeted nature of MFFFA include:

1 Neurological damage resulting from delayed diagnosis of vitamin B12 deficiency which is most commonly prevalent in the elderly. It is estimated that 5% of the US population aged 50 and above exceed the UL for folic acid (54).

2 The uncertain considerations of long-term novel folic acid intakes especially for children facing a lifetime of increased intake. It is estimated that 4% of Australian children exceed the UL for folic acid (55).

3 Lingering concerns about possible influence of folic acid in promoting the progression of pre-existing colorectal cancer.

The degree of quality control with MFFFA's implementation has a bearing on risk. The practice of overage (adding additional amounts of a fortificant to a food) has been observed to occur with folic acid in a number of countries, raising concerns that a greater proportion of the population may exceed the UL than was predicted. Soon after MFFFA was implemented in the US it was observed that fortification was occurring at twice mandated levels and not accurately reflected on food labels (56) and was matched with raised blood folic acid levels. This situation was subsequently controlled after monitoring findings were published (57). In Canada MFFFA has also been observed to have been implemented with the addition of folic acid to some foods at 50% higher than mandated levels and not reflected in product labels (58).

Secondary risk There are no secondary risks.

Practical disadvantages MFFFA is indiscriminate in its action. The MFFFA intervention needs to be designed so that it delivers an adequate but not excessive dose of folic acid to the target group while not delivering an excessive amount of folic acid to the population as a whole. This explains its risks and adverse ethical considerations.

Ethical considerations

Effectiveness MFFFA is consistently reported as an effective policy option. It cannot account for all risk factors for NTDs but in most countries where it has been implemented it has been estimated to reduce NTD prevalence by 20–56%.

Proportionality Although NTDs are especially tragic and cause severe malformations, they have a low prevalence across the population, especially in relation to conventional micronutrient malnutrition problems for which mandatory food fortification is recommended. Therefore is it proportional that for each NTD prevented several hundred thousand people are exposed, without choice, to extra folic acid? (59). The answer will vary depending on from whose perspective this question is viewed.

As a population-wide policy intervention MFFFA is not a proportional policy option. All infants, children, men, and older adults who consume fortified foods will have an increased intake of folic acid for no apparent benefit and with possible risk, and often without their knowledge. Commonly, public health policy interventions are justified on the grounds of proportionality, even if they might place some individuals at modest risk, so long as they provide sufficient benefit for the population as a whole. This perspective is captured in the utilitarian approach of doing 'the greatest good for the greatest number'. MFFFA as a policy option to decrease NTD prevalence represents the opposite of the utilitarian approach. MFFFA is increasing the folic acid intake, and potential risk, of the many in order to increase the folic acid intake, and likely benefit, of susceptible women who may become pregnant.

As a policy intervention for genetically susceptible women MFFFA is a proportional policy option. The potential risks of excessive folic acid intake are far outweighed by the reduced risk of having an NTD-affected pregnancy.

Necessity MFFFA is not necessary. Alternative policy options to MFFFA are available to help reduce the risk of NTDs. Indeed, the dosage used in many countries may be insufficient to reach the recommended intake and hence other options are required in parallel. For this reason some countries that have recommended MFFFA also recommend that folic acid supplements be consumed. For example the US Preventive Services Task Force recommends that all women planning or capable of pregnancy take a daily supplement containing 400–800 µg of folic acid (60). If a daily folic acid supplement is recommended regardless of MFFFA and the minimum dose of folic acid in the supplement can be prescribed to achieve the recommended folic acid intake, the need for MFFFA is redundant.

Least infringement MFFFA is the most coercive of the policy options available to reduce the risk of NTDs. It indiscriminately increases the folic acid intake of everyone in the population who consumes the fortified staple food(s). This indiscriminate delivery raises fundamental ethical concerns. In particular, is it appropriate to expose everyone in the population to raised levels of synthetic folic acid, for the benefit of a relatively small number of individuals? This ethical concern is exacerbated in the context that this raised exposure will provide no apparent benefit to the majority of the population and may be associated with potential risks as it is difficult for authorities to implement the policy without exposing certain population groups to levels of folic acid above the UL and there remain questions about whether it promotes colorectal cancer.

Public justification There is little evidence that MFFFA has been complemented with substantial public justification. Policy decisions typically are made with minimal public consultation and once implemented the presence of folic acid in staple foods is not obvious to the public as it does not overtly affect the taste or presentation of foods. Public justification depends indirectly on the coexistence of promotion activities for alternative policy options such as supplementation and it is rare in such instances that the public is advised about the passive exposure, scientific uncertainties and ethical considerations of MFFFA. Although researchers have often surveyed the target group to assess its awareness and understanding of MFFFA, far less surveillance has engaged the remainder of the population to assess its awareness, understanding and attitude towards MFFFA.

Voluntary flour fortification with folic acid

Description

Voluntary fortification with folic acid arises when decisions about if and when fortification with folic acid might take place, what food vehicle is used, and at what level of fortification, are determined by food manufacturers. Food products such as breakfast cereals have been voluntarily fortified with folic acid for a number of years. This policy option is particularly common in Europe.

Relationship of this policy option to the cause of the policy problem

Voluntary flour fortification with folic acid does not directly address the cause of the policy problem.

Public health benefits

In many countries there is available a variety of foods voluntarily fortified with folic acid, especially cereals. The advantages of a policy intervention that promotes the availability of these foods is that it will raise the background exposure of folic acid to at-risk individuals and it provides choice to those individuals who do not need or want to be exposed to high levels of folic acid.

Ireland provides some important insights in relation to this policy option. In 1980, the NTD rate in Ireland was approximately five per 1000 births, while for the rest of Europe rates were estimated as being around 1.2 per 1000 births (61). One explanation of this rate differential was that termination of pregnancy is illegal in Ireland and relative to many other countries a high number of NTD-affected pregnancies are carried to full term and delivered as live births. In 2006 the Irish Minister for Health and Children accepted the recommendation of the National Committee on Folic Acid Food Fortification to introduce a programme of mandatory folic acid fortification of bread (62).

Yet, the Irish population has one of the highest per capita consumptions of fortified breakfast cereals (63). In 2008, the Irish Department of Health and Children was advised by the Food Safety Authority of Ireland that the target population was obtaining sufficient folate from their diets due to an escalation in the number of voluntarily folic acid-fortified food products in the marketplace (64). The Department was also advised that this raised folic acid intake had resulted in an observed increase in red cell folate levels among the population and a fall in the rate of NTD birth prevalence (65). The following year the Food Safety Authority of Ireland announced that it had put its previous policy recommendation on hold. The Authority explained that the increased availability of folic acid in the food supply since the original mandatory folic acid fortification recommendation had been made and the incidence of NTDs having been reduced to 0.93 per 1000 live births, meant that there would be limited public health benefit from introducing mandatory folic acid fortification at that time (66).

For those countries that have introduced MFFFA it is no longer possible to distinguish the contribution of voluntarily fortified foods to the folic acid intakes and evaluate their impact on NTD rates. In Australia the NTD incidence rate (1.09 per 1000 pregnancies) was estimated immediately before the introduction of MFFFA as part of a baseline report for future evaluation of the policy. The report also revealed that in the ten years leading up to the baseline estimate, a period coinciding closely with the introduction of voluntary folic acid fortification in Australia, the NTD incidence rate had decreased by 26% (55). These data indicate that as Australia's NTD rate is already approaching the 'floor' of minimum NTD rates that might be achieved from increased folic acid intakes the MFFFA policy may be operating on diminishing returns.

Public health risks

Primary risk Excessive folic acid intake though the risk is less than that for MFFFA as there is less folic acid present in the food supply.

Practical disadvantages The policy option's implementation is at the discretion of food manufacturers for whom the protection and promotion of public health cannot be expected to be a primary responsibility. Hence, it is difficult for policy-makers to predict which food products might be fortified with folic acid, when, and at what levels, and therefore to be confident that there will be an adequate and consistent folic acid exposure in the food supply.

Ethical considerations

Unlike MFFFA, voluntary food fortification with folic acid provides individuals with a choice to purchase non-folic acid fortified food products.

Folic acid supplementation

Description

Folic acid supplementation can be delivered in the form of folic acid tablets or multivitamin tablets containing folic acid. The dose recommendation varies among countries but typically ranges from 400–500 µg for women of childbearing age and 4–5 mg for women who previously have had a NTD-affected pregnancy.

Relationship of this policy option to the cause of the policy problem

Folic acid supplementation relates directly and efficiently to the presumed cause of the policy problem. Supplements can be selected with a dosage to match the recommended intake level to compensate for the presumed genetic polymorphism affecting folate metabolism. The supplement can be targeted efficiently to at-risk individuals without increasing the folic acid intake of other individuals or the population as a whole.

Public health benefits

Effectiveness In ideal circumstances folic acid supplementation would be expected to achieve a 70% reduction in recurrence and 62% reduction in occurrence of NTDs based on a meta-analysis of experimental and observational studies (46). This evidence of supplementation efficacy, obtained from the controlled environment of research trials, represents an 'upper ceiling' to which supplementation interventions conducted in the real world might strive.

In practice it is reported that globally less than half of the target group take periconceptional folic acid supplements (67). In countries around the world the effectiveness of folic acid supplementation as a policy option varies with the circumstances and presence of complementary strategies with which it is implemented. Particularly impressive results have been reported for interventions that are targeted through primary health care settings. For example, in 1995 the Dutch government sponsored a national mass media campaign to promote folic acid supplement usage by women planning a pregnancy.

The campaign was attributed with achieving a 33% reduction in NTD prevalence in the years 1996–1999 to 2000–2002 (68). Then in 2004 Dutch pharmacies began a campaign aimed at motivating women using oral contraceptives to take folic acid supplements before conception and it has been reported that in 2005, 51% of respondents in the target group used folic acid supplements throughout the periconceptional period (69). In areas of China the evaluation of intensive promotion campaigns delivered in health care settings has reported even higher levels of compliance (70). A critical characteristic in both these evaluations has been a high percentage of planned pregnancies among the populations where the intervention was carried out, e.g. in the Netherlands almost 80% of pregnancies are planned, well above the European average (69). Nevertheless, elsewhere where unplanned pregnancies are more common similar findings have been reported. A US trial involving the provision of free folic acid supplements to patients during routine gynaecological visits reported a 68% increase in folic acid intake among the intervention group (including a large proportion of disadvantaged individuals not planning pregnancies) compared with 20% in the control (71). The characteristic in common across these three successful interventions has been the intensive involvement of the primary health care sector.

Cost-effectiveness There have been few studies that have evaluated the cost-effectiveness of folic acid supplementation. A study commissioned by Food Standards Australia New Zealand during its consideration of MFFFA concluded that folic acid supplementation in combination with voluntary folic acid fortification was more cost-effective than MFFFA (72).

Equity In their review of supplementation interventions from 1989 to 2006 in Europe, USA, Canada, Australia and New Zealand, Stockley and Lund report only modest compliance of the target group with supplementation recommendations and disadvantaged women within the group were least compliant (73) suggesting a significant gap in NTD prevalence reduction from the ideal. This disparity has been shown to persist in a situation of relatively high compliance when 51% compliance of the target group was observed, and the behaviour was reported by 63% of the higher-educated women and just 31% of the less-educated women (69). This disparity in compliance with folic acid supplementation recommendations is of concern because NTDs have a higher prevalence in low socioeconomic and less educated groups relative to more advantaged groups.

Practical advantages The practical advantages of supplementation are that the dose of folic acid can be precisely set to the recommended level for the target group and the intervention can be targeted to at-risk individuals and not the wider population.

Public health risks

Primary risk Excessive folic acid intake is rare but can occur as a result of excessive (dose/frequency) supplement consumption.

Practical disadvantages The supplementation policy option requires an ongoing investment to sustain awareness and motivation among the target group and to inform women who newly enter childbearing years.

Ethical considerations

Effectiveness Low-high effectiveness depending on investment in complementary strategies.

Proportionality Supplementation is a proportional policy option as the benefits it provides to at-risk individuals outweigh the potential risks of excessive folic acid intake and it is not targeted at populations.

Necessity Supplementation is not the only option that might decrease NTD prevalence, but if it is not recommended in its own right it is usually recommended as a complement to other policy options.

Least infringement Supplementation is a low infringement policy option as individuals can choose whether or not to consume supplements.

Public justification Supplementation needs to be complemented with public education approaches to promote compliance and to inform at risk individuals about potential benefits and risks.

Nutrition education

Description

Nutrition education refers to the provision of programmes and materials designed to raise the public's awareness and skills in selecting, preparing and consuming a healthy diet containing folate-rich foods.

Relationship of this policy option to the cause of the policy problem

Nutrition education as described in this investigation does not relate directly to the cause of the policy problem as its purpose is to promote a healthy balanced diet consistent with dietary guideline messages designed for the general population and not at-risk individuals with raised nutrient requirements.

Public health benefits

Not all of the experimental trials and observational studies that contributed to the evidence base that informed the original MFFFA policy recommendations were based on folic acid intake. One of those important early studies was a case-control study that reported that dietary folate was an independent risk factor for NTDs (74). Nevertheless, policy recommendations are expressed in terms of folic acid intake and the assumption has been that nutrition education is not a feasible policy option because it is too difficult for the target group to consume a sufficient amount of the less bioavailable folate through the diet to achieve the recommended folic acid intake level. Conversely, others such as Nestle have argued that recommended intake levels can be achieved through folate rich diets (75). Additionally, a large US study reported that a healthy balanced maternal diet in the year before pregnancy was associated with lower risks for NTDs and orofacial clefts (cleft palate) suggesting that overall diet quality may be predictive of birth defect risk (76). However, others have shown that policy interventions promoting fruit and vegetables as food folate sources have yielded poor success (77).

Nutrition education has the secondary public health benefit of promoting a healthy diet to improve the overall nutritional health of the target group and population.

Public health risks

There are no public health risks.

Ethical considerations

Nutrition education has modest evidence of effectiveness as a stand-alone policy option; it has minimal infringement and is a proportional policy option in the sense that there are no substantive risks to negate the potential benefit. However, it is most clearly ethically justified when implemented as a complement to alternative policy options as it informs the target group and population of the policy problem.

Maintaining the status quo

Description

Maintaining the status quo refers to deliberately deciding to not respond to epidemiological evidence for the folic acid–NTD relationship.

Relationship of this policy option to the cause of the policy problem

No relationship to the cause of the policy problem.

Public health benefits

This policy option provides policy-makers with time to observe the implications of other NTD prevention policy options being implemented elsewhere. However, there will be no public health benefits from deciding to not respond

Table 6.1 Summary of public health benefits, risks, and ethical considerations of policy options available to respond to the epidemiological evidence for the folic acid—NTD relationship

Policy option	Public health benefit	Public health risk	Ethical considerations
Mandatory flour fortification with folic acid	Low–high effectiveness	Moderate risk of excessive intake and subsequent masking of neurological symptoms of vitamin B12 deficiency	Low ethical justification
	Mixed evidence of cost-effectiveness		Not proportional—a non-targeted approach of high benefit for at-risk individuals but affecting the whole population for little benefit and possible risk.
	Equitable		
	Does not require behaviour change	Lingering concerns about risk of promoting the progression of colorectal cancer	High coercion
	A secondary benefit is that in those countries with folate deficiency MFFFA will increase folic acid intake to help prevent anaemia.		Not necessary
	A practical advantage is that the government has control over timing, levels and extent of fortification	A practical disadvantage is that MFFFA is indiscriminate in its delivery of folic acid	Not publicly justified
Voluntary flour fortification with folic acid	Low–high effectiveness	Low-moderate risk of excessive intake for the population and the target group	As for MFFFA though less effective and less coercive—more free choice for individuals
	Limited evidence of cost-effectiveness		
		The food industry is responsible for implementation so difficult to control timing, level and extent of fortification	

Folic acid supplementation	Low–high effectiveness Some evidence of cost-effectiveness Low equity Advantage of delivering direct to target group Can deliver a precise minimum dose	No risk for the population Low risk of excessive intake for the target group Practical disadvantage that effectiveness is dependent on behaviour change and ongoing compliance	High ethical justification High proportionality–high benefit for at-risk individuals and low risk for population Low infringement on the population and maintains individuals' free choice Necessary Publicly justified
Nutrition education	Low–modest effectiveness Limited evidence of cost-effectiveness Low equity Secondary benefits in promoting a healthy diet for target group and population	Practical disadvantage of requiring a significant change in current dietary behaviours to achieve folic acid intake recommendations	Low effectiveness for the target group Maintains individuals' free choice Necessary in that it informs the target group and the population about the policy problem and complements alternative policy options
Maintaining the status quo	Not effective, cost-effective or equitable Has the practical advantage of providing policy-maker with time to obtain more evidence	Nil NTD prevalence will return to pre-intervention levels if an effective policy option is stopped.	Represents a precautionary approach ('First do no harm') and maintains population's free choice Not proportional or necessary as there exists convincing evidence

to the epidemiological evidence for reducing the risk of NTDs because there will be no increase in folic acid intake to prevent NTD-affected pregnancies.

Public health risks

There are no public health risks associated with a decision to maintain the status quo as there is no policy intervention. When an effective NTD risk reduction policy option is stopped the prevalence of NTDs will return to pre-intervention levels.

Ethical considerations

Maintaining the status quo is the policy option which infringes the least on individuals and the population but it fails to meet the other four 'justificatory conditions'. In the context of the scientific uncertainties and potential risks it might be argued that it is an ethically justified policy option because it is upholding the Hippocratic oath of first doing no harm. However, given the convincing evidence of the folic acid–NTD relationship this policy option is not a proportional response when there are other policy options available that can moderate risk, albeit with less benefit.

Analysing the policy process: chronology of the making of MFFFA policy

1990s

The impetus for policy-makers to consider MFFFA was the publication of the findings from trials reporting the protective effect of folic acid supplements for the occurrence (32) and recurrence of NTDs (31) in the early 1990s. Shortly after these studies were published, the CDC recommended that all women of childbearing age consume 400 µg of folic acid daily to help prevent NTDs (78). Similar recommendations followed shortly thereafter in many countries around the world. Commonly, this involved recommending a 0.4 mg folic acid supplement daily to all women planning pregnancy and 4 mg folic acid to those with a previous NTD-affected pregnancy. Voluntary folic acid fortification was permitted in many countries at this time and in some countries where it was not permitted the regulations were reviewed so that staple foods could be fortified with the intention of increasing the availability of folic acid in the food supply, albeit at food manufacturers' discretion (79).

There was public, professional, and political debate in many countries during the mid-1990s about how best to respond to the epidemiological evidence for the folic acid–NTD relationship. Although some initially questioned the quality of the evidence, most of the debate focused on what was the preferred policy response. Complicating the debate in several countries was its intertwining with another vexed food policy debate—the use of health claims on food labels and in food marketing that were prohibited at that time (75). Health claims are those claims that describe a relationship between a food and a health effect, such as 'food product X can help reduce the risk of heart disease'. Removing the prohibition to enable the use of such claims for marketing purposes was a goal of many food manufacturers. In 1995 the Kellogg Company and the March of Dimes, (the mission of the latter is 'to improve the health of babies by preventing birth defects, infant mortality, and premature birth') (80) jointly developed a folic acid health message for placement on Kellogg's Product 19 (81). A related development in Australia in 1998 involved the Health Minister speaking at a Kellogg's Nutrition Summit in which he referred to the need to review the existing prohibition on health claims and that the folic acid–NTD health message needs to be communicated (82). Subsequently a folic acid–NTD health claim that linked consumption of a folic acid-rich food with a reduced risk of NTDs was devised (83). This health claim was established as a pilot project and created the exception to the existing prohibition on health claims in Australia. The appeal to food manufacturers was that it opened the door slightly on the existing prohibition on health claims. The appeal to food regulators was that an increased amount of folic acid would be available in the food supply. Curiously, a subsequent evaluation revealed that although food manufacturers did add folic acid to a wider range of their products only two of an eligible 128 products used the health claim (84).

In 1996 Oman became the first country to implement MFFFA when it approved the addition of 5 mg/kg folic acid to white flour as a policy option to prevent NTDs (85). It achieved this status by happening to be in the midst of a trial testing the feasibility of flour fortification when a regional workshop on health interventions was held. Oman was able to respond to the discussions by scaling up its trial to broader national coverage (86). In the same year the US FDA issued regulations requiring all 'enriched' cereal grain products be fortified with folic acid at 140 μg/100 g cereal grain by 1 January 1998 (87).

2000s

The impetus that the US MFFFA regulations created gave momentum for this policy option to be considered in many other countries, e.g. they provided a template for technical considerations such as the level of folic acid fortification. Over the next 16 years, national recommendations for MFFFA spread steadily throughout Latin and South America, the Middle East, and parts of Africa and the Western pacific.

During the 2000s there were also significant developments to secure support for MFFFA on the international stage. In 2004 the FFI, the CDC, and the

Mexican Institute of Public Health jointly convened in Cuernavaca, Mexico a technical workshop entitled 'Wheat Flour Fortification: Current Knowledge and Practical Applications', (88). The workshop was supported by the CDC, March of Dimes, MI, and GAIN. Four years later the FFI hosted its Second Technical Workshop on 'Wheat Flour Fortification: Practical Recommendations for National Application' in Georgia, USA to provide advice for countries considering national wheat and/or maize flour fortification (45). The technical papers presented at the workshop endorsed MFFFA as well as other food fortification policies. The steering committee for this workshop consisted of representatives from among other agencies, the CDC, MI, GAIN, FFI, and WHO. The following year the WHO issued a consensus statement endorsing fortification of flour with iron, folic acid, vitamin B12, vitamin A, and zinc (6). This guideline was prepared by the core group from WHO's Department of Nutrition for Health and Development in close collaboration with the Food and Agriculture Organization, the nutrition section of UNICEF, GAIN, MI, and FFI. The WHO commented that the guideline was based on scientific reviews prepared for the FFI technical workshop held in Stone Mountain, GA, USA in 2008.

2010s

In 2010 a special supplement of the *Food and Nutrition Bulletin*, entitled, 'Flour fortification with iron, folic acid, vitamin B12, vitamin A, and zinc: Proceedings of the Second Technical Workshop on Wheat Flour Fortification' (89) was published and it again drew from the technical background documents that were presented at the FFI technical workshop held in Stone Mountain, GA, USA in 2008. The supplement repeated the technical workshop's call for MFFFA. Later in 2010, the Sixty-third World Health Assembly and the 126th session of the Executive Board adopted a number of resolutions and decisions in relation to birth defects (90). The World Health Assembly urged Member States to increase coverage of folic acid supplementation and requested the Director-General support Member States in developing national plans for implementation of food fortification strategies, for the prevention of birth defects, and promoting equitable access to such services.

As at 2012, 66 countries have recommended MFFFA as national policy—mostly in wheat flour and within the range 100–300 μg/100 g (91). It is not always possible to ascertain if the primary motivation for MFFFA recommendations has been NTD prevention or as a conventional food fortification policy responding to evidence of population-wide folate deficiency. Several countries (Ireland, New Zealand, UK) initially did recommend MFFFA but subsequently expressed concerns about their original recommendation and have since either reversed or deferred their recommendation. Also, the US is reviewing its

MFFFA policy to consider increasing the number of food products mandated to be fortified with folic acid.

Discussion

The public health benefits, risks and ethical considerations of MFFFA

MFFFA is associated with mixed public health benefits and risks and has a low ethical justification. Evaluative evidence consistently indicates that it is effective in helping prevent NTDs though the level of effectiveness varies with the baseline NTD prevalence, the national frequency of the 677 TT polymorphism, proportion of unplanned pregnancies and folate status of the target group. It is equitable as it has the practical advantage of passively increasing the folic acid intake of everyone who consumes products made from fortified flour. Paradoxically, its key practical advantage in achieving effectiveness and equity—that it passively exposes the target group to increased folic acid—is also its key disadvantage in that it indiscriminately exposes everyone in the population to novel levels of a synthetic vitamin for the rest of their lives.

The indiscriminate nature of MFFFA exposes this policy option to concerns about its public health risks. Some have likened its action in increasing the population's folic acid intake to it being a form of 'uncontrolled clinical trial' (92). In a similar vein, while acknowledging its effectiveness but equally drawing attention to its public health risks, others have described the policy as a 'double-edged sword' (93). The ethical justification for MFFFA is weak as assessed against the five principles in this investigation. It is not proportional at the population level, it is not necessary, it has a high level of infringement and rarely has been publicly justified.

The assessment of public health benefits, risks and ethical considerations varied among the four alternative policy options. Relative to these alternative policy options with which it was compared MFFFA was generally more positively assessed for public health benefits. An exception being the special case of preventing recurrent NTDs for which supplementation was the most effective and equitable as the necessary 4–5-mg dose could be made available and intended recipients would be aware of the need to consume the supplement. One qualifier in comparing the relative public health benefits of the alternative policy options is that they have not been evaluated to the same extent as MFFFA for their effectiveness and cost-effectiveness in reducing NTD prevalence. All of the policy alternatives were associated with less public health risk than MFFFA. The ethical justification for all of the alternative policy options was stronger than for MFFFA.

The primary lesson from the assessment of this case study was the critical importance of matching a potential policy option to the underlying cause of a policy problem. The degree of alignment of a potential policy option with the underlying cause of NTDs was predictive of the extent of public health benefit, risk and ethical considerations. This was demonstrated by the positive findings for supplementation which was the policy option most directly responding to the aetiological evidence for NTDs (Figure 6.2).

The assessment for this case study was unable to account for variations in local circumstances among countries. Countries with relatively high NTD rates, low folate status (especially if associated with anaemia), high national frequency of the *MTHFR* C677T polymorphism and high proportion of unplanned pregnancies, are likely to achieve a higher reduction in NTD prevalence (and anaemia prevention) from MFFFA than other countries. These differential impacts will have a bearing on the assessment of public health benefits, risks and ethical considerations associated with each policy option for a particular country.

The policy process for MFFFA

Presented with the same epidemiological evidence, policy-makers in countries around the world have interpreted this evidence in different ways to formulate different policy responses. It is a highly contested and controversial public

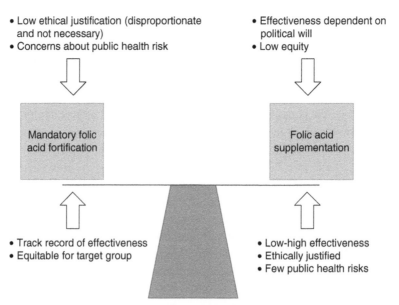

- Low ethical justification (disproportionate and not necessary)
- Concerns about public health risk

- Effectiveness dependent on political will
- Low equity

Mandatory folic acid fortification

Folic acid supplementation

- Track record of effectiveness
- Equitable for target group

- Low-high effectiveness
- Ethically justified
- Few public health risks

Fig. 6.2 The major pros and cons of mandatory flour fortification with folic acid versus folic acid supplementation in preventing NTDs.

health policy topic. There are geographical clusters of countries that have recommended MFFFA and these include the Americas, the Middle East, parts of Africa, and the Western Pacific. There are other geographical clusters where MFFFA has not been recommended, most notably Europe where a diversity of voluntarily folic acid fortified food products are available and promotion campaigns have been implemented, albeit usually on a short-term basis.

Few policy-makers question the epidemiological evidence for the folic acid–NTD relationship. Instead the political debate is about to which policy option should this evidence be interpreted as supporting. The complicating circumstances associated with NTDs set up the policy-making process to confront some major evidential and ethical challenges in judging how best to translate the epidemiological evidence into a policy solution. In this regard MFFFA is a particularly rich case study to observe how and why food fortification policy is made. In this section, a description of how and why MFFFA is being promoted at the international level is provided. There are many actors within countries and globally who are involved in activities to promote MFFFA. A brief description of the role and influence of the more prominent global actors as identified in the earlier chronology of MFFFA developments is presented along with examples of their activities in promoting MFFFA and the relevant agendas within which food fortification policy-making is operating.

Actors

This description of the more prominent global actors is structured around their sophisticated advocacy for MFFFA and their network of interactions with other actors.

The US Centers for Disease Control and Prevention (CDC) In 1992 it was the CDC that was among the first agencies to recommend that all women of childbearing age consume 400 µg of folic acid daily to help prevent NTDs (78). Around this time the CDC, through the then Director of its Division of Birth Defects and Developmental Disabilities, Dr Godfrey Oakley, along with the March of Dimes, began advocating for folic acid to be added to the US standard for enriched flour (94). It continues to be highly supportive of MFFFA, describing it as one of the ten great public health achievements in the US during the decade 2001–2010 (95).

Now the CDC's National Center on Birth Defects and Developmental Disabilities has developed a 'Global Initiative to Eliminate Folic Acid-Preventable Neural Tube Defects'. The aim of the initiative is to expand the number of low- and middle-income countries (LMICs) with mandatory folic acid fortification of 'high penetrance staples' and among its strategic objectives are to work with the WHO and others 'to establish a global policy to support and advance country-level fortification efforts (96).

The CDC has been a nurturer of many of the prominent global actors involved in promoting MFFFA. In 2004 it contributed to the formation of the FFI (97) and it continues to fund FFI's global secretariat as well as serving as a member of the FFI Executive Management Team (97). Dr Godfrey Oakley has gone on to become one of the strongest advocates for MFFFA internationally. In addition, the current Coordinator of WHO Micronutrient's Division, previously worked at the CDC where he was actively involved in the monitoring and evaluation of flour fortification programmes (98).

Flour Fortification Initiative (FFI) FFI is the world's leading advocate for MFFFA. Formed in 2004, it is a network of public, private, and civic organizations that is working towards making fortification of wheat flour a standard practice globally. FFI's goal is for '80% of the world's roller miller flour to be fortified with at least iron or folic acid by 2015' (45). It has a well-developed and resourced strategy (99) that guides it in working with national leaders to advocate for flour fortification, provide technical assistance and resources for putting fortification plans into practice, and to undertake monitoring and surveillance of performance against objectives. It has been very effective in placing MFFFA on the political agenda internationally with its series of technical workshops in the 2000s and in promoting recommendations to engage in MFFFA in many countries. FFI lists among its partners the CDC, MI, GAIN and the WHO.

Micronutrient Initiative (MI) MI has been a strong supporter of both MFFFA and folic acid supplementation activities especially in Bangladesh, India and Nepal (100). In 2003 it was the prime mover in establishing a coalition of international organizations to advocate for worldwide action on increasing folic acid uptake to prevent NTDs (101). It is involved in partnerships with FFI, GAIN and the WHO to promote MFFFA.

GAIN GAIN's goal is to reach 1.5 billion people with fortified foods including foods fortified with folic acid (102). It is pursuing this goal with partnerships with the CDC, MI, FFI and the WHO and the private sector and is heavily supported by the Bill & Melinda Gates Foundation and USAID, amongst others at lesser levels.

Champions for MFFFA advocacy An important advocacy strategy is to have a champion who can represent the face of an advocacy programme by appearing in the media, meeting with policy-makers and engaging in public, professional and political debate for an issue. Champions need to be committed to the issue, well networked and especially energetic in prosecuting a case. MFFFA has attracted a range of champions around the world. The most energetic champion has been Professor Godfrey Oakley who has been described as the 'folic acid ambassador' for his advocacy role in encouraging countries to fortify flour with folic acid (45). When Director of the CDC's Division of Birth Defects and Developmental Disabilities, he joined with the March of Dimes to advocate for folic acid to be added to the US standard for enriched flour that then led to the US issuing this regulation in 1996. He has published many articles in professional journals advocating for MFFFA. In addition to his connections with CDC, in his current role as research professor of epidemiology at the Rollins School of Public Health at Emory University, he is linked with the FFI whose website has been hosted by this university.

WHO

The WHO's support for MFFFA is strong and represented in its 2009 Recommendations on wheat and maize flour fortification (6). The WHO receives grants from MI, CDC and GAIN for this programme, and is actively engaged in partnerships with these organizations as well as FFI. As noted earlier, the Coordinator of WHO Micronutrient's Division, Dr Juan Pablo Pena-Rosas, previously worked at CDC as an expert in monitoring flour fortification. In 2011 he was appointed as an Adjunct Assistant Professor at the Rollins School of Public Health at Emory University in the US where Professor Godfrey Oakley is based and where the FFI website has been hosted.

These actors are influential and well-resourced advocates for MFFFA as the preferred policy option to help prevent NTDs. There are no equivalent actors who overtly advocate on the international stage for alternative policy options to help prevent NTDs. There is a degree of 'push-back' questioning MFFFA in the scientific press, especially from European work, though this does not have the same advocacy impact. The actors present a strong united front complementing each other's activities. As depicted in Figure 6.3 they participate in a network of interactions so as to form an effective coalition to advocate for MFFFA.

Activities

Advocacy has been a core activity in policy-making processes for MFFFA around the world. The influence of advocacy in shaping national MFFFA recommendations is described with reference to experiences in New Zealand and Fiji.

New Zealand—duelling advocacy campaigns and the MFFFA rollercoaster
In the mid-2000s New Zealand was reviewing the policy options available to respond to the epidemiological evidence of the folic acid–NTD relationship. At that time the NTD birth prevalence was relatively low by international

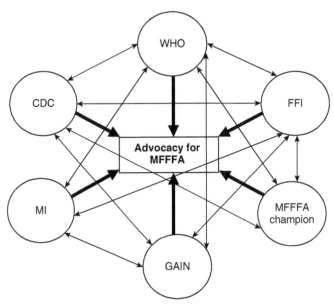

Fig. 6.3 The coalition of global advocates for mandatory folic acid fortification and their network of interactions.

standards at approximately 6 per 10,000 (103). Also at that time, foods including bread and breakfast cereals were permitted to be voluntarily fortified with folic acid and were widely available.

Activities undertaken by the FFI and civil society advocates contributed to the country's regulatory agency recommending MFFFA as the preferred policy option in 2007 (104). It was estimated that this policy would reduce the number of NTD-affected pregnancies by 4–14 cases (up to 20% of the total cases). However, during the two-year-phase in period for the policy an advocacy campaign undertaken by the baking industry, and in combination with a change in government, resulted in the policy being deferred until 2012 (105). The change in policy position frustrated advocates for MFFFA with an FFI report commenting that 'Sheep blocking a road on the South Island in New Zealand symbolize the roadblocks faced in attempting to implement mandatory flour fortification in Ireland and New Zealand' (106). Further advocacy by FFI and civil society organizations again contributed to mandatory MFFFA being positioned as the proposed policy option by the New Zealand Ministry for Primary Industries in 2012 (107).

In the five-year period 2007–2012, New Zealand has experienced a MFFFA policy rollercoaster—recommending, deferring and then finally choosing to reject this policy (108). The evidence to inform the policy has not changed significantly during this period. Instead the alternating policy positions reflect duelling advocacy campaigns by actors for and against MFFFA.

Fiji—the role of advocacy in MFFFA policy-making in the absence of evidence The following example of advocacy to regulate MFFFA in a country is taken from a review (109) of the policy development process associated with regulating MFFFA in Fiji.

Advocacy for flour fortification in Fiji began in the late 1980s. Fiji, along with most Pacific Island countries, does not have a strong capacity to undertake comprehensive nutrition monitoring and surveillance activities. Nevertheless, there was available at that time substantial evidence of significant and persistent iron deficiency anaemia among the Fijian population to support the case for mandatory iron fortification of flour. Evidence to support mandating other nutrient fortification was not available. According to the review, in 1999 a UNICEF consultant undertook an assessment of the feasibility of iron fortification for Fiji and although he only reviewed the case for iron-deficiency anaemia, he recommended that wheat flour be fortified not just with iron but also zinc, folic acid, thiamin, riboflavin and niacin. The justification for recommending MFFFA was that it had been introduced in the US as a policy option to decrease NTD prevalence and that flour fortification offered an opportunity to add other micronutrients by using standard premixes. In 2000 the Fijian Cabinet agreed that the Ministry of Health should proceed with flour fortification. Since 2004, Fiji has required all flour to be fortified with the micronutrients recommended by the consultant in 1999. This country example highlights that advocacy can be effective in bringing about the regulation of MFFFA despite the absence of evidence of a population's folic acid consumption, folic acid status and NTD prevalence rates. Instead the rationale was opportunistic, i.e. the flour was already being fortified with iron, so it was decided to extend the fortification to include other nutrients regardless of there being no evidence available to support such an approach. This lack of evidence to inform folic acid fortification is not unique to Fiji. The WHO Executive Board has noted that the magnitude of folate deficiency and folate status at national level for many countries is poorly known (110). Of relevance to the MFFFA policy decision in Fiji are study findings from countries in the Western Pacific region. The findings indicate that following education and social socioeconomic levels, will purchase and consume vitamin supplements (111).

Framing has been a significant strategy as a complement to the advocacy for MFFFA. NTDs are devastating and the need to prioritize their prevention generates much emotion in policy discussions. MFFFA variously has been described as a 'miracle' (112) and a policy that urgently needs attention (113). Some have gone so far as to state that governments who delay introducing MFFFA are committing 'public health malpractice' (114).

One common feature of MFFFA framing has been to accentuate its benefits, e.g. claiming that this policy option will prevent up to 70% of NTD cases (even in countries with a high folate status and low NTD prevalence) (115). Others claim that MFFFA can reduce the risk of other birth defects (6) despite there being no statistically significant evidence to support this claim (33). Proponents often frame MFFFA as a simple, straightforward policy decision with almost all 'up-side' and little if any 'down-side'. For example, FFI and CDC are essentially as one in presenting the case for MFFFA when they state, 'The need is abundant, the strategy is effective, the costs are low, and the potential benefit is staggering' (45) *and* 'Fortification of flour and other high-consumption, high-penetration staples with folic acid is a feasible, economical, safe, and effective public health policy to prevent NTDs worldwide' (97).

A second common feature of MFFFA framing is to diminish concerns about its risks and ethical considerations. Some advocates directly tackle concerns by stating outright that fortification of wheat flour with folic acid is safe (45). Others shift the blame for excessive folic acid intakes and potential adverse effects in populations away from MFFFA and on to folic acid supplement use (116). In Germany (117) and Canada (118) scientists have recommended that regulations be introduced to limit the use and marketing of such supplements. Elsewhere risks linked to MFFFA such as masking the symptoms of vitamin B12 deficiency are often described as 'theoretical' and by inference dismissed as being of concern. Such inferences overlook the existence of a UL based on such risks and, irrespective of one's view about the risks, it is a dubious approach to be advocating for a policy if it knowingly increases the proportion of the population who exceed the UL.

A powerful form of framing relates to what is not presented in policy forums, in other words, framing by omission. The aetiological evidence for underlying cause(s) of NTDs is often not presented in policy forums. This situation means that there is lacking a frame of reference to understand public health risks and ethical considerations associated with different policy options. Complicating circumstances have necessarily framed the policy response as needing to be directed at a target group and not targeted at genetically predisposed women. However, this can confuse understanding of this topic; with some believing NTDs to be caused by a conventional population-wide folate deficiency rather than individuals within that group having an increased folic acid requirement. For example, MI does not differentiate between NTDs and anaemia when stating that both can result from folic acid deficiency (100). Yet they are distinct—NTDs most commonly result from a failure of at-risk individuals to meet an increased folic acid requirement whereas anaemia most commonly has a population-wide prevalence resulting from folate (and not folic acid) deficiency. The distinction is important because it has a bearing on assessing public health benefits, risks and ethical considerations of different policy options.

Agendas

Global health governance The global health governance agenda around PPPs has facilitated the ability of certain actors to gain privileged access to the UN system and to participate in key policy-making developments to promote MFFFA. The WHO's involvement with PPPs has seen it actively engaged with CDC, FFI, MI, and GAIN in policy discussions that preceded and then included its 2009 Recommendations on wheat and maize flour fortification (6). The Recommendation's Report acknowledges that the WHO Micronutrients Unit receives grants from MI, CDC, and GAIN, among others. The report explains clearly that donors do not fund specific guidelines and do not participate in any decision related to the guideline development process.

International food trade International food trade has not been an explicit influence on the MFFFA policy debate. The one notable exception arose immediately following the US decision to recommend MFFFA. Originally Canadian food regulators did not support MFFFA and urged the US FDA to not proceed with their MFFFA proposal. However, Canadian flour millers were not prepared to produce different flours for the domestic and US markets and they applied the political pressure that led Health Canada to recommend MFFFA for Canada (119).

The analysis of this case study indicates that the policy-making process associated with MFFFA internationally displays characteristics in common with all three political science theoretical frameworks reviewed in Chapter 2 (multiple streams, advocacy coalition framework (ACF) and network approach). In particular, characteristics of the policy-making can be described to a significant degree by drawing on features outlined in the ACF approach. When policy options have been recommended, a strong predictor of MFFFA has been the combination of actors, activities and agendas working in concert. Powerful actors with a shared belief in MFFFA as the preferred policy option have operated both independently and as part of a coalition of actors. They have been the dominant coalition in the absence of an alternative coalition with different beliefs towards policy options—those who believe in alternative policy options have operated more as individuals. The coalition has undertaken sophisticated and persistent advocacy to influence key events and policy outcomes. The way that evidence of benefits and risks of policy interventions to decrease NTD prevalence has been framed has been instrumental in explaining how scientific uncertainties and ethical dilemmas have been rationalized. The global health governance agenda seeking out PPPs has elevated the influence of these advocacy coalitions by facilitating their access to UN agencies and key policy-making forums.

The advocacy for MFFFA can be compelling for governments wanting to be seen to be acting on the epidemiological evidence. MFFFA is attractive because it is a relatively straightforward policy response that can achieve demonstrable change in the target group and population's folate status relatively quickly. In contrast, alternative policy options such as supplementation require more sophisticated approaches and a sustained investment to achieve similar changes in folate status. Some stress that this attractiveness is understandable but because of the complexity of folic acid–health relationships care must be taken so that policy decisions are based on scientific evidence rather than 'political expediency' (93).

In their analysis of the MFFFA policy debate in Australia and New Zealand, Begley and Coveney conclude that a biomedical frame of reference dominated how MFFFA was represented in the media and professional journals. They comment that this observation reflected the traditional power and influence of the medical profession in framing the debate and influencing the policy process and the ultimate decision to recommend MFFFA (120).

The dominant role of medical views in shaping public health policy has been understood for many years (121). What is unusual with the findings from this case study is that the exertion of the medical views is in a reverse orientation to that normally observed. Rather than advocacy focusing on the use of a medical intervention to help solve a public health problem as occurs when a nutrient supplement is proposed to correct a population-wide nutrient deficiency, in this case study a public health intervention is being appropriated to help solve a medical problem.

This description of how and why MFFFA has been adopted does not extend to cases where MFFFA has not (yet) been recommended. This is not to suggest that a decision to not recommend MFFFA is apolitical. Political processes and activities such as advocacy and framing can be just as relevant in explaining how and why a food fortification policy is made as well as how and why it is not made. However, there is a not an equivalent set of actors or extent of activities being undertaken, or agendas that are combining to promote supplementation or voluntary food fortification, in the way that these variables have come together to promote MFFFA internationally.

A national food regular's recommendation for or against MFFFA reflects its judgement on the public health benefits, risks and ethical considerations of policy options. For some countries such as the UK concerns about public health risks have explained its policy response. In 2006, the Scientific Advisory Committee on Nutrition (SACN) that advises the UK Food Standards Agency and the UK Department of Health recommended that MFFFA should proceed (122). Then a year later in response to emerging evidence, the Chief Medical Officer requested advice from SACN on potential adverse effects of folic acid on colorectal cancer risk (123). In 2009, the SACN agreed that there were uncertainties but concluded that there were insufficient data to support the concerns that folic acid fortification promoted cancer and re-confirmed its previous recommendation for MFFFA (123). In noting that approximately 106,000 people in the UK were exceeding the UL for folic acid it also recommended voluntary controls on folic acid supplement and voluntary folic acid fortified food marketing and consumption be implemented. The UK government is yet to implement such voluntary controls or regulate MFFFA.

After initially recommending MFFFA, the Food Safety Agency of Ireland re-assessed their decision when evidence was provided indicating that voluntary folic acid fortification permissions were sufficient to achieve the folic acid policy recommendations. Similarly in Finland, it was decided that a relatively low NTD rate and the contribution of folate from the diet and voluntarily fortified foods made the requirement for MFFFA redundant (124). In New Zealand the government's 2007 decision to regulate MFFFA was deferred shortly before it was to come into effect in 2009. After investing resources in advocating for MFFFA in New Zealand, the FFI undertook an analysis of the reason for this deferral (106). Its analysis concluded that the deferral of the New Zealand government's MFFFA recommendation was primarily the result of an advocacy campaign coordinated by local bakers and supported by a new government that was elected during the phase in period for the MFFFA regulation.

The different circumstances of high-income countries (HICs) and LMICs provide a point of difference to explain why some countries do or don't recommend MFFFA. In LMICs, the less developed primary health care delivery systems and the relatively higher cost of supplements for populations with less disposable income presents more challenges for the supplementation policy option relative to MFFFA. At the same time the substantial prevalence of conventional folate deficiency-disease outcomes in LMICs such as anaemia, may displace NTDs as the primary folate related policy problem needing attention. In this situation the policy debate becomes far more complex, as multiple policy options need to be considered for multiple folate-related policy problems.

Future directions for preventing NTDs

Folic acid supplementation (as opposed to fortification) was used in the original clinical trials in the early 1990s that established the convincing epidemiological evidence for the protective effect of folic acid in reducing the risk of NTDs. Into the future there is a strong case for this policy option being preferred for NTD prevention programmes. It is the policy option that most closely aligns with the cause of NTDs, it has the potential for the greatest reduction in NTD prevalence, it has a low level of public health risk and it is ethically justified. The primary constraint on folic acid supplementation's acceptance is its reliance on political will. Whereas many governments have stated their commitment to NTD prevention they rarely have matched such statements with sufficient and sustained investment in folic acid supplementation promotion to enable it to achieve its full potential (125, 126). Novel approaches to supplementation offer another opportunity to increase compliance. For example, the addition of folate in the form of metafolin or tetrahydrofolate to oral contraceptives is showing promise (127). Though seemingly counterintuitive, this approach has the advantages of being directed at the target group, it can be complemented with information to increase awareness for when contraception is discontinued, and as oral contraceptives are routinely not taken as prescribed, unplanned pregnancy rates can be significant.

There is important research that still needs to be conducted to address the existing scientific uncertainties associated with the folic acid–NTD relationship. If the mechanism by which folic acid reduces the risk of NTDs could be elucidated, scientists would be closer to being able to design a screening tool to identify at-risk women, as well as gaining a greater understanding of the precise dose and timing, for folic acid to deliver a maximum protective effect. Ongoing research into the potential benefits and risks of folic acid for the target group and population as a whole will also help inform policy-making for NTD prevention. Given folate's role in many important biochemical pathways there is much potential for additional benefits and risks to be identified with novel ways to increase the intake of this nutrient. Overall, this is a dynamic area with folic acid regularly linked to a variety of health outcomes. Should it be demonstrated that folic acid intake is related to the protection or promotion of a major disease such as cardiovascular disease then the assessment equation for MFFFA would need to be urgently re-addressed.

The aetiological evidence for NTDs suggests that they are caused by a combination of environmental and genetic factors, and that increased folic acid intake may prevent up to 70% of cases. This means that even if an ideal folic acid intake were to be achieved, 30% of NTD cases would persist. Other policy interventions will be required for their prevention.

Monitoring and evaluation is a priority for future NTD prevention interventions. Previously concerns have been expressed that systems for monitoring

MFFFA have not been adequate (128). For example, many countries have commenced their implementation of MFFFA without adequate baseline measures being put in place to inform later evaluation. It is not just the impact of MFFFA on NTD rates that is important, more evidence on the relative effectiveness, cost-effectiveness and equity implications of all policy options is required to better inform policy-making.

Monitoring of policy options also needs to be vigilant for additional public health benefits and risks that might arise for the target group and the wider population (129). However, this presents a peculiar challenge. It can be predicted that as a consequence of MFFFA, the folic acid intakes of populations will be at novel levels and for novel periods of time (children will be exposed to a lifetime of raised levels of folic acid). It cannot be predicted what might be the impact of such novel intake patterns on public health benefits and risks, especially for a nutrient as metabolically influential as folic acid. In this situation, drawing on knowledge of the basic biological pathways with which folate is involved will help researchers anticipate where potential health outcomes might arise. A further challenge for monitoring and evaluation activities is that it will be difficult to detect potential benefits and risks of policy options because already there exists background exposure to folic acid, and in the case of MFFFA, there is no unexposed comparison group (130). One research group unable to demonstrate a relationship between folic acid and stroke prevention have suggested that this outcome may be reversed if they were to repeat their study with a population that was not exposed to MFFFA (131).

Lessons from the case study findings for the food fortification rationale

Adding a nutrient(s) to food to compensate for certain individuals having nutrient requirements higher than reference standards was proposed as one of three rationales for mandatory food fortification (Chapter 1, Table 1.1). In this section the case study findings are generalized to identify lessons regarding the plausibility of this particular food fortification rationale.

The case study findings indicate that MFFFA was associated with mixed public health benefits and risks and adverse ethical considerations. There are limitations in using food fortification as a policy solution for a policy problem that it is presumed is caused predominantly by a genetic polymorphism. Also, MFFFA is not relevant for addressing other NTD causes that account for approximately 30% of risk. NTDs are a peculiar policy problem in that complicating circumstances provide a reason for MFFFA to be considered as a policy solution. Nonetheless the observations from assessing and analysing MFFFA as a policy solution for NTDs indicate that it does not provide a strong case for accepting certain individuals having a nutrient requirement above reference standards as a rationale for food fortification.

There is another policy problem that falls within this food fortification rationale—micronutrient malnutrition when it is caused by a parasitic infection or a related medical condition in individuals, e.g. anaemia caused by worms and blood loss. Here food fortification, in the form of iron fortification of flour, could provide additional iron to help meet the raised iron requirement of affected individuals. In this situation, food fortification is not addressing the underlying cause of the policy problem, instead it is treating the symptoms. Based on the findings from this present case study (which also did not address the underlying cause of the problem) it would be predicted that the food fortification policy option may have limited public health benefits, some public health risks, and low ethical justification. In addition, and unlike the situation with NTDs, there is no apparent complicating circumstance that warrants its special consideration. However unlike NTDs, anaemia caused by parasitic infections and related conditions can be highly prevalent across populations. This situation would result in greater ethical justification for food fortification within this rationale especially as a temporary or complementary solution until a policy option that directly and sustainably treats the underlying cause of the problem is implemented.

The case study has raised the following ethics-related questions to consider when assessing whether 'certain individuals having nutrient requirements above reference standards' is a plausible rationale for food fortification:

1 What level of disease severity and prevalence resulting from a medical condition in individuals justifies food fortification?

   NTDs are severe congenital malformations in certain individuals but fortunately they are not prevalent across the population. Anaemia resulting from parasitic infections and related conditions may not be as severe as NTDs but it is substantially more prevalent in some countries. Currently there are no guidelines on what level of disease severity and prevalence resulting from a medical condition in individuals justifies food fortification.

2 When formulating MFFFA interventions what proportion of a population exceeding the UL is acceptable?

   A core challenge for formulating the technical conditions associated with MFFFA is that the policy needs to achieve a population folic acid consumption profile that fits within the narrow window of exposure that is both effective and safe. Whereas the target group needs to consume an additional 400 µg folic acid/day, the population as a whole needs to consume no more than 1mg folic acid/day to avoid exceeding the UL for this nutrient. In several countries that are implementing MFFFA it is estimated that 4–5% of the population is exceeding the UL of folic acid intake. Is it appropriate to maintain a policy intervention that is known to be responsible for this degree of excessive folic acid intake? Currently there are no guidelines for judging what proportion of the population exceeding the UL should be tolerated.

Conclusion

MFFFA as a policy option to decrease NTD prevalence has created a precedent for mandating the fortification of food. It was and remains the only example where mandatory food fortification has been recommended based on the rationale of adding a nutrient to a food(s) to help meet the predominantly genetically-mediated raised nutrient requirements of certain individuals, rather than tackling a population-wide nutrient deficiency. For this reason MFFFA is a complex and controversial policy option for decreasing NTD prevalence. The application of food fortification in this instance is not without reason. There is no policy option available to efficiently target all women who are genetically predisposed to having an NTD-affected pregnancy. In those countries where MFFFA has been recommended as the policy option in response to this peculiar situation, it generally has been effective in preventing almost one-half of NTD cases and usually in an equitable fashion.

Nevertheless, this novel application of mandatory food fortification—it is being co-opted to serve a medical treatment role—creates a precarious situation. MFFFA is delivering a synthetic form of a natural vitamin in relatively high amounts to the target group and it is doing so in an indiscriminate way so that everyone who consumes the fortified staple food(s) will have an increased intake of folic acid. For infants, children, men and older adults, this raised folic acid intake will occur without apparent benefit and often without their knowledge. MFFFA is not a policy option that efficiently addresses the underlying cause of the policy problem. Public health risks are evident and it is a struggle to justify this policy option against the ethical principles adopted in this investigation. Overall, the observations from this case study do not provide strong support for mandatory food fortification when the rationale for adding nutrients to food is that certain individuals have nutrient requirements higher than reference standards.

The need to formulate a policy response in the context of scientific uncertainties, ethical dilemmas and complicating circumstances has brought many political dynamics to the surface. It has provided a valuable opportunity to how and why epidemiological evidence is translated into food fortification policy. There are five potential policy responses to the epidemiological evidence.

In many of those countries where MFFFA has been recommended, it is evident that a medical view towards food and health relationships has dominated policy-making as a result of a compelling combination of powerful actors undertaking sophisticated advocacy and supported by global health governance agendas.

More than 20 years after the convincing epidemiological evidence that folic acid reduces the risk of NTDs was published approximately one-third of countries around the world have adopted MFFFA. Also during this period, few governments have invested substantially and sustainably in alternative policy options. The exciting prospect is that there is the potential for governments to do much more to reduce NTD prevalence if the political will exists for greater investment in alternative policy options such as folic acid supplementation interventions involving primary health care delivery services. Evaluations of this option have shown promising outcomes with the possibility of achieving levels of NTD prevention comparable with MFFFA while being associated with less public health risk and problematic ethical considerations. There remain many unknowns. Based on this case study's findings, adding nutrients to foods to compensate for certain individuals having nutrient requirements above reference standards is a problematic rationale for mandatory food fortification policy and practice.

References

1. Darnton-Hill I, Mora J, Weinstein H, Wilbur S, Nalubola P. Iron and folate fortification in the Americas to prevent and control micronutrient malnutrition: an analysis. *Nutrition Reviews* 1999; 57(1):25–31.
2. Christianson A. Howson CP, Modell B. *The March of Dimes Global Report on Birth Defects: The Hidden Toll of Dying and Disabled Children.* New York: March of Dimes Birth Defects Foundation; 2006. [cited 7 May 2012]. Available from: http://www.marchofdimes.com/downloads/Birth_Defects_Report-PF.pdf.
3. Wald N. Folic acid and the prevention of neural tube defects. *Annals of the New York Academy of Sciences* 1993; 678:112–29.
4. Goldacre B. *Bad Science.* London: Fourth Estate; 2008, pp. 152–3.
5. Rosenberg I. Folic acid fortification. *Nutrition Reviews* 1996; 54(3):94–5.
6. World Health Organization. *Recommendations on wheat and maize flour fortification meeting report: interim consensus statement.* 2009 [cited 28 March 2012]. Available from: http://www.who.int/nutrition/publications/micronutrients/wheat_maize_fortification/en/index.html.
7. Wills L. Treatment of 'pernicious anaemia of pregnancy' and 'tropical anaemia'. *British Medical Journal* 1931; 1(3676):1059–64.
8. Hoffbrand AV, Weir DG. The history of folic acid. *British Journal of Haematology* 2001; 113(3):579–89.
9. Cornel MC, de Smit DJ, de Jong-van den Berg LT. Folic acid—the scientific debate as a base for public health policy. *Reproductive Toxicology* 2005; 20(3):411–15.

10. Stover PJ. Folate biochemical pathways and their regulation. In: Bailey LB (ed). *Folate in Health and Disease*, 2nd ed. Gainesville, FL: CRC Press, Taylor & Francis Group; 2009, pp. 49–74.

11. Cavelaars AE, Doets EL, Dhonukshe-Rutten RA, Hermoso M, Fairweather-Tait SJ, Koletzko B, *et al.* Prioritizing micronutrients for the purpose of reviewing their requirements: a protocol developed by EURRECA. *European Journal of Clinical Nutrition* 2010; 64(Suppl 2):S19–30.

12. Kalmbach RD, Choumenkovitch SF, Troen AM, D'Agostino R, Jacques PF, Selhub J. Circulating folic acid in plasma: relation to folic acid fortification. *American Journal of Nutrition* 2008; 88(3):763–8.

13. Sweeney MR, Staines A, Daly L, Traynor A, Daly S, Bailey SW, *et al.* Persistent circulating unmetabolised folic acid in a setting of liberal voluntary folic acid fortification. Implications for further mandatory fortification? *BMC Public Health* 2009; 9:295–301.

14. Smith R. Let food be thy medicine. *British Medical Journal* 2004; 328:180.

15. Israels M, Wilkinson J. Risk of neurological complications in pernicious anaemia treated with folic acid. *British Medical Journal* 1949 (ii):1072–5.

16. Institute of Medicine of the National Academies. *Dietary reference intakes for thiamin, riboflavin, niacin, vitamin B6, folate, vitamin B12, pantothenic acid, biotin, and choline.* Washington, DC: Institute of Medicine of the National Academies; 2000, pp. 150–95.

17. Kallen B. Use of folic acid supplementation and risk for dizygotic twinning. *Early Human Development* 2004; 80(2):143–51.

18. Kiefte-de Jong JC, Timmermans S, Jaddoe VW, Hofman A, Tiemeier H, Steegers EA et al. High circulating folate and vitamin B-12 concentrations in women during pregnancy are associated with increased prevalence of atopic dermatitis in their offspring. *J Nutr* 2012; 142:731–38.

19. Whitrow MJ, Moore VM, Rumbold AR, Davies MJ. Effect of supplemental folic acid in pregnancy on childhood asthma: a prospective birth cohort study. *American Journal of Epidemiology* 2009; 170(12):1486–93.

20. Morris M, Jacques P, Rosenberg I, Selhub J. Folate and vitamin B-12 status in relation to anemia, macrocytosis, and cognitive impairment in older Americans in the age of folic acid fortification *American Journal of Clinical Nutrition* 2007; 85(1):193–200.

21. Walker JG, Batterham PJ, Mackinnon AJ, Jorm AF, Hickie I, Fenech M, *et al.* Oral folic acid and vitamin B-12 supplementation to prevent cognitive decline in community-dwelling older adults with depressive symptoms—the Beyond Ageing Project: a randomized controlled trial. *American Journal of Nutrition* 2012; 95(1):194–203.

22. Kim Y-I. Folic acid fortification and supplementation – good for some but not so good for others. *Nutrition Reviews* 2007; 65(11):504–11.

23. Ebbing M, Bonaa KH, Nygard O, Arnesen E, Ueland PM, Nordrehaug JE, *et al.* Cancer incidence and mortality after treatment with folic acid and vitamin B12. *Journal of the American Medical Association* 2009; 302(19):2119–26.

24. Mason J, Dickstein A, Jacques P, Haggarty P, Selhub J, Dallal G, *et al.* A temporal association between folic acid fortification and an increase in colorectal cancer rates may be illuminating important biological principles: a hypothesis. *Cancer Epidemiology Biomarkers and Prevention* 2007; 16(7):1325–9.

25. Stevens V, McCullough M, Sun J, Jacobs E, Campbell P, Gapstur S. High levels of folate from supplements and fortification are not associated with increased risk of colorectal cancer. *Gastroenterology* 2011; 141(1):98–105.

26. Kennedy D, Stern S, Moretti M, Matok I, Sarkar M, Nickel C, *et al.* Folate intake and the risk of colorectal cancer: a systematic review and meta-analysis. *Cancer Epidemiology* 2011; 35(1):2–10.

27. Lee JE, Willett WC, Fuchs CS, Smith-Warner SA, Wu K, Ma J, *et al.* Folate intake and risk of colorectal cancer and adenoma: modification by time. *American Journal of Nutrition* 2011; 93(4):817–25.

28. Gibson TM, Weinstein SJ, Pfeiffer RM, Hollenbeck AR, Subar AF, Schatzkin A, *et al.* Pre- and postfortification intake of folate and risk of colorectal cancer in a large prospective cohort study in the United States. *American Journal of Nutrition* 2011; 94(4):1053–62.

29. Mason J. Folate consumption and cancer risk: a confirmation and some reassurance, but we're not out of the woods quite yet *American Journal of Clinical Nutrition* 2011; 94(4):965–6.

30. Hibbard ED, Smithells, RW. Folic acid metabolism and human embryopathy. *Lancet* 1965; 285:1254.

31. Medical Research Council Vitamin Study Research Group. Prevention of neural tube defects: Results of the Medical Research Council Vitamin Study. *Lancet* 1991; 338:131–7.

32. Czeizel A, Dudas I. Prevention of the first occurrence of neural-tube defects by periconceptional vitamin supplementation. *New England Journal of Medicine* 1992; 327:1832–5.

33. De-Regil LM, Fernandez-Gaxiola AC, Dowswell T, Pena-Rosas JP. Effects and safety of periconceptional folate supplementation for preventing birth defects. *Cochrane Database of Systematic Reviews* 2010; 10:CD007950.

34. Dary O. Nutritional interpretation of folic acid interventions. *Nutrition Reviews* 2009; 67(4):235–44.

35. Heseker H, Mason J, Selhub J, Rosenberg I, Jacques P. Not all cases of neural-tube defect can be prevented by increasing the intake of folic acid. *British Journal of Nutrition* 2009; 102(2):8.

36. Ray JG, Wyatt PR, Vermeulen MJ, Meier C, Cole DE. Greater maternal weight and the ongoing risk of neural tube defects after folic acid flour fortification. *Obstetrics and Gynecology* 2005; 105(2):261–5.

37. Grewal J, Carmichael SL, Song J, Shaw GM. Neural tube defects: an analysis of neighbourhood- and individual-level socio-economic characteristics. *Paediatric and Perinatal Epidemiology* 2009; 23(2):116–24.

38. Molloy AM, Brody LC, Mills JL, Scott JM, Kirke PN. The search for genetic polymorphisms in the homocysteine/folate pathway that contribute to the etiology of human neural tube defects. *Birth Defects Research Part A: Clinical and Molecular Teratology* 2009; 85(4):285–94.

39. Botto LD, Yang Q. 5,10-methylenetetrahydrofolate reductase gene variants and congenital anomalies: a HuGE review. *American Journal of Epidemiology* 2000; 151:862–77.

40. Esfahani ST, Cogger EA, Caudill MA. Heterogeneity in the prevalence of methylenetetrahydrofolate reductase gene polymorphisms in women of different ethnic groups. *Journal of the American Dietetic Association* 2003; 103(2):200–7.

41. Cotter AM, Daly SF. Neural tube defects: is a decreasing prevalence associated with a decrease in severity? *European Journal of Obstetrics, Gynecology, and Reproductive Biology* 2005; 119(2):161–3.

42. Wald NJ, Law MR, Morris JK, Wald DS. Quantifying the effect of folic acid. *Lancet* 2001; 358(9298):2069–73.

43. Moore LL, Bradlee ML, Singer MR, Rothman KJ, Milunsky A. Folate intake and the risk of neural tube defects: an estimation of dose-response. *Epidemiology* 2003; 14(2):200–5.

44. Han JY, Nava-Ocampo AA, Koren G. Unintended pregnancies and exposure to potential human teratogens. *Birth Defects Research Part A: Clinical and Molecular Teratology* 2005; 73(4):245–8.

45. Flour Fortification Initiative [cited 28 September 2012]. Available from: http://www.ffinetwork.org/.

46. Blencowe H, Cousens S, Modell B, Lawn J. Folic acid to reduce neonatal mortality from neural tube disorders. *International Journal of Epidemiology* 2010; 39(Suppl 1):110–21.

47. Calvo EB, Biglieri A. Impact of folic acid fortification on women's nutritional status and on the prevalence of neural tube defects. *Archivos Argentinos de Pediatría* 2008; 106(6):492–8.

48. Williams LJ, Rasmussen SA, Flores A, Kirby RS, Edmonds LD. Decline in the prevalence of spina bifida and anencephaly by race/ethnicity: 1995–2002. *Pediatrics* 2005; 116(3):580–6.

49. Barboza Arguello Mde L, Umana Solis LM. Impact of the fortification of food with folic acid on neural tube defects in Costa Rica. *Revista Panamericana de Salud Pública* 2011; 30(1):1–6.

50. Grosse SD, Waitzman NJ, Romano PS, Mulinare J. Reevaluating the benefits of folic acid fortification in the United States: economic analysis, regulation, and public health. *American Journal of Public Health* 2005; 95(11):1917–22.

51. Bentley TG, Weinstein MC, Willett WC, Kuntz KM. A cost-effectiveness analysis of folic acid fortification policy in the United States. *Public Health Nutrition* 2009; 12(4):455–67.

52. Sumar N, McLaren L. Impact on social inequalities of population strategies of prevention for folate intake in women of childbearing age. *American Journal of Public Health* 2011; 101(7):1218–24.

53. U.S. Centers for Disease Control and Prevention. CDC grand rounds: additional opportunities to prevent neural tube defects with folic acid fortification. *Morbidity and Mortality Weekly Report* 2010; 59(31):980–4.

54. Bailey RL, Dodd KW, Gahche JJ, Dwyer JT, McDowell MA, Yetley EA, *et al.* Total folate and folic acid intake from foods and dietary supplements in the United States: 2003–2006. *American Journal of Nutrition* 2010; 91(1):231–7.

55. Australian Institute of Health and Welfare. *Mandatory folic acid and iodine fortification in Australia and New Zealand: supplement to the baseline report for monitoring.* Cat. no. PHE 153. Canberra: AIHW. 2011.

56. Rader J, Weaver CM, Angyal G. Total folate in enriched cereal-grain products in the United States following fortification. *Food Chemistry* 2000; 70:275–89.

57. Johnston KE, Tamura T. Folate content in commercial white and whole wheat sandwich breads. *Journal of Agricultural and Food Chemistry* 2004; 52(20): 6338–40.

58. Shakur YA, Rogenstein C, Hartman-Craven B, Tarasuk V, O'Connor DL. How much folate is in Canadian fortified products 10 years after mandated fortification? *Canadian Journal of Public Health* 2009; 100(4):281–4.

59. Smith AD. Folic acid fortification: the good, the bad, and the puzzle of vitamin B-12. *American Journal of Nutrition* 2007; 85(1):3–5.

60. U.S. Preventive Services Task Force. Folic Acid for the Prevention of Neural Tube Defects: U.S. Preventive Services Task Force Recommendation Statement U.S. Preventive Services Task Force. *Annals of Internal Medicine* 2009; 150:626–31.

61. Abramsky L, Busby A, Dolk H. Promotion of periconceptional folic acid has had limited success. *Journal of the Royal Society for the Promotion of Health* 2005; 125(5):206–9.

62. National Committee on Folic Acid Food Fortification. *Report of the National Committee on Folic Acid Food Fortification*. Dublin: Food Safety Authority of Ireland; 2006.

63. Fletcher RJ, Bell IP, Lambert JP. Public health aspects of food fortification: a question of balance. *Proceedings of the Nutrition Society* 2004; 63(4):605–14.

64. Food Safety Authority of Ireland. *Report of the Implementation Group on Folic Acid Food Fortification to the Department of Health and Children*. [cited 1 October 2010]. Available from: http://www.fsai.ie/WorkArea/DownloadAsset.aspx?id=7602.

65. Flynn M, Anderson W, Burke S, Reilly A. Session 1: public health nutrition. Folic acid food fortification: the Irish experience. *Proceedings of the Nutrition Society* 2008; 67(4):381–9.

66. Food Safety Authority of Ireland. *Currently no need for mandatory fortification— increased folate status negates mandatory folic acid fortification at this time*. [cited 1 October 2010]. [Press release]. Available from: http://www.fsai.ie/news_centre/press_releases/11032009.html.

67. Ray JG, Singh G, Burrows RF. Evidence for suboptimal use of periconceptional folic acid supplements globally. *BJOG: an international journal of obstetrics and gynaecology* 2004; 111(5):399–408.

68. de Jong-van den Berg LT. Monitoring of the folic acid supplementation program in the Netherlands. *Food and Nutrition Bulletin* 2008; 29(Suppl):S210–3.

69. de Walle H, de Jong-van den Berg L. Ten years after the Dutch public health campaign on folic acid: the continuing challenge. *European Journal of Clinical Pharmacology* 2008; 64(5):539–43.

70. Berry RJ, Li Z, Erickson JD, Li S, Moore CA, Wang H, *et al*. Prevention of neural-tube defects with folic acid in China. China-U.S. Collaborative project for neural tube defect prevention. *New England Journal of Medicine* 1999; 341(20):1485–90.

71. Robbins JM, Cleves MA, Collins HB, Andrews N, Smith LN, Hobbs CA. Randomized trial of a physician-based intervention to increase the use of folic acid supplements among women. *American Journal of Obstetrics and Gynecology* 2005; 192(4): 1126–32.

72. Dalziel K, Segal L, Katz R. Cost effectiveness of mandatory folate fortification v. other options for the prevention of neural tube defects: results from Australia and New Zealand. *Public Health Nutrition* 2010; 13(4):566–78.

73. Stockley L, Lund V. Use of folic acid supplements, particularly by low-income and young women: a series of systematic reviews to inform public health policy in the UK. *Public Health Nutrition* 2008; 11(8):807–21.

74. Bower C, Stanley FJ. Dietary folate as a risk factor for neural-tube defects: evidence from a case-control study in Western Australia. *Medical Journal of Australia* 1989; 150(11):613–19.

75. Nestle M. Folate fortification and neural tube defects: policy implications. *Journal of Nutrition Education* 1994; 26(6):287–93.

76. Carmichael SL, Yang W, Feldkamp ML, Munger RG, Siega-Riz AM, Botto LD, *et al.* Reduced risks of neural tube defects and orofacial clefts with higher diet quality. *Archives of Pediatric & Adolescent Medicine* 2012; 166(2):121–6.

77. Busby A, Abramsky L, Dolk H, Armstrong B. Preventing neural tube defects in Europe: population based study. *British Medical Journal* 2005; 330(7491):574–5.

78. U.S. Centers for Disease Control and Prevention. Recommendations for the use of folic acid to reduce the number of cases of spina bifida and other neural tube defects. *MMWR Morbidity and Mortality Weekly Report* 1992; 41:1–7.

79. National Health and Medical Research Council. *NHMRC revised statement on the relationship between dietary folic acid and neural tube defects such as spina bifida.* 1993.

80. March of Dimes. *History.* [cited 15 May 2012]. Available from: http://www.marchofdimes.com/mission/history_qa.html.

81. Anon. Kellogg and March of Dimes develop folate health message for product 19. *Food Labeling News* 1995; June 22, p. 15.

82. Australia New Zealand Food Authority. *ANZFA media news* 1998; 18 March Canberra: Australia New Zealand Food Authority; 1998.

83. Australia New Zealand Food Authority. *An Interim Code of Practice for the communication of the health benefits of food products to be used in a pilot for health claims relating to folate/neural tube defects 1998–1999 was approved.* Canberra: Australia New Zealand Food Authority; 1998.

84. Lawrence M. Evaluation of the implementation of the folate-neural tube defect health claim and its impact on the availability of folate-fortified food in Australia. *Australian and New Zealand Journal of Public Health* 2006; 30(4):363–8.

85. Alasfoor D, Elsayed M, Mohammed A. Spina bifida and birth outcome before and after fortification of flour with iron and folic acid in Oman. *Eastern Mediterranean Health Journal* 2010; 16(5):533–38.

86. Zimmerman S. Fifteen years of fortifying with folic acid: birth defects are reduced and healthcare expenses are averted. *Sight and Life* 2011; 25:54–9.

87. US Food and Drug Administration. Food standards: amendment of standards of identity for enriched grain products to require addition of folic acid. *Federal Register* 1996; 61(4):8781–97.

88. Flour Fortification Initiative. *Report of the Workshop of Wheat Flour Fortification.* Cuernavaca: Flour Fortification Initiative, 2004 [cited 13 May 2010]. Available from: http://www.sph.emory.edu/wheatflour/CKPAFF/index.htm.

89. Serdula M, Peña-Rosas JP, Maberly GF, Parvanta I. *Flour fortification with iron, folic acid, vitamin B12, vitamin A, and zinc: Proceedings of the Second Technical Workshop on Wheat Flour Fortification. Food and Nutrition Bulletin* 2010; 31(Suppl 1). [cited 13 May 2010]. Available from: http://nsinf.publisher.ingentaconnect.com/content/nsinf/fnb;jsessionid=hcpdc577vs2n.alice.

90. World Health Assembly. Resolution WHA63.17. Birth defects. In: *Sixty-third World Health Assembly, Geneva 17–21 May 2010. Resolutions and decisions.* Geneva: World Health Organization; 2010.

91. Lawrence M, Kripalani K. Profiling national mandatory folic acid fortification policy around the world. In: Preedy V (ed). *Handbook of food fortification and health: from concepts to public health applications.* New York: Springer; in press.

92. Skeaff M, Green T, Mann J. Mandatory fortification of flour? Science, not miracles, should inform the decision. *New Zealand Medical Journal* 2003; 116(1168):U303.

93. Lucock M, Yates Z. Folic acid fortification: a double-edged sword. *Current Opinion in Clinical Nutrition and Metabolic Care* 2009; 12(6):555–64

94. Flour Fortification Initiative. *Fifteen years of fortifying with folic acid reduces birth defects; averts healthcare expenses.* [cited 13 May 2012]. Available from: http://www.sph.emory.edu/wheatflour/FortifyForLifeBackground.pdf.

95. U.S. Centers for Disease Control and Prevention. Ten great public health achievements—United States, 2001–2010. *Morbidity and Mortality Weekly Report* 2011; 60(19):619–23. [cited 6 May 2012]. Available from: http://www.cdc.gov/mmwr/preview/mmwrhtml/mm6019a5.htm?s_cid=mm6019a5_w.

96. U.S. Centers for Disease Control and Prevention. *Global initiative to eliminate folic acid-preventable neural tube defects.* [cited 29 May 2012]. Available from: http://www.cdc.gov/ncbddd/folicacid/global.html.

97. U.S. Centers for Disease Control and Prevention. CDC grand rounds: additional opportunities to prevent neural tube defects with folic acid fortification. *Morbidity and Mortality Weekly Report* 2010; 59(31):980–4. Available from: http://www.cdc.gov/mmwr/preview/mmwrhtml/mm5931a2.htm.

98. Pena-Rosas JP, Parvanta I, van der Haar F, Chapel TJ. Monitoring and evaluation in flour fortification programs: design and implementation considerations. *Nutrition Reviews* 2008; 66(3):148–62.

99. Flour Fortification Initiative. [cited 19 March 2012]. Available from: http://www.sph.emory.edu/wheatflour/strategy.php.

100. Micronutrient Initiative. *Folic acid* [cited 5 October 2012]. Available from: http://www.micronutrient.org/English/View.asp?x=581.

101. Oakley G, Bell K, Weber M. Recommendations for accelerating global action to prevent folic acid-preventable birth defects and other folate-deficiency diseases: meeting of experts on preventing folic acid-preventable neural tube defects. *Birth Defects Research Part A: Clinical and Molecular Teratology* 2004; 70(11):835–7.

102. Global Alliance for Improved Nutrition. *About GAIN.* 2011 [updated 2011; cited 23 March 2012]. Available from: http://www.gainhealth.org/about-gain.

103. The Center of the International Clearinghouse for Birth Defects Surveillance and Research. *Annual Report 2008 with data for 2006.* Roma: International Clearinghouse for Birth Defects Surveillance and Research; 2008.

104. Food Standards Australia New Zealand. *First Review Report, Proposal P295, Consideration of Mandatory Fortification with Folic Acid.* 2007. [cited 26 May 2012]. Available from: http://www.foodstandards.gov.au/_srcfiles/P295%20Folate%20Fortification%20FFR%20+%20Attach%201%20FINAL.pdf.

105. TvNZ. *Voluntary folate in bread wins day. TVNZ.* 2009. [cited 5 October 2012]. Available from: http://tvnz.co.nz/politics-news/voluntary-folate-in-bread-wins-day-2949599.

106. Flour Fortification Initiative. *Roadblocks to progress: a look at why Ireland and New Zealand halted mandatory flour fortification with folic acid.* [cited 26 May 2012]. Available from: http://www.sph.emory.edu/wheatflour/IrelandNewZealand.pdf.

107. Ministry for Primary Industries. *The future of folic acid fortification of bread in New Zealand,* MPI Discussion Paper No: 2012/02, May 2012. [cited 26 May 2012]. Available from: http://www.foodsafety.govt.nz/elibrary/industry/fortification-bread-folic-acid/folic-acid-discussion-document.pdf.

108. Ministry for Primary Industries. *Scientific evaluation of comments on submissions received on the future of folic acid fortification in New Zealand.* [cited 26 September 2012]. Available from: http://www.foodsafety.govt.nz/elibrary/industry/fortification-bread-folic-acid/index.htm.

109. Snowdon W. *Legislation to mandate the supply of fortified flour in Fiji Desktop Review of Policy development process.* Suva, Fiji: National Food and Nutrition Centre; 2011.

110. World Health Organization. *Executive Board EB130/11, 130th session 20 December 2011, Provisional agenda item 6.3 Nutrition, Nutrition of women in the preconception period, during pregnancy and the breastfeeding period.* Report by the Secretariat. Geneva: WHO; 2011.

111. Cavalli-Sforza T, Berger J, Smitasiri S, Viteri F. Weekly iron-folic acid supplementation of women of reproductive age: impact overview, lessons learned, expansion plans, and contributions toward achievement of the millennium development goals. *Nutrition Reviews* 2005; 63(12 Pt 2):S152–8.

112. Oakley G, Wald N, Omenn G. Provide the citizens of New Zealand the miracle of folic acid fortification. *New Zealand Medical Journal* 2003; 116(1168):U302.

113. Maberly GF, Stanley FJ. Mandatory fortification of flour with folic acid: an overdue public health opportunity. *Medical Journal of Australia* 2005; 183(7):342–3.

114. Oakley GP. Delaying folic acid fortification of flour: Governments that do not ensure fortification are committing public health malpractice. *British Medical Journal* 2002; 324(7350):1348–9.

115. Stanley FJ. *Failure to fortify with folate condemns hundreds of children to debilitating birth defects.* [Media release] Subiaco: Telethon Institute for Child Health Research; 2006.

116. Berry RJ, Bailey L, Mulinare J, Bower C. Fortification of flour with folic acid. *Food and Nutrition Bulletin* 2010; 31(Suppl 1):S22–35.

117. Herrmann W, Obeid R. The mandatory fortification of staple foods with folic acid: a current controversy in Germany. *Deutsches Ärzteblatt International* 2011; 108(15):249–54.

118. Shakur YA, Garriguet D, Corey P, O'Connor DL. Folic acid fortification above mandated levels results in a low prevalence of folate inadequacy among Canadians. *American Journal of Nutrition* 2010; 92(4):818–25.

119. Oakley GP, Jr. Folate deficiency is an 'imminent health hazard' causing a worldwide birth defects epidemic. *Birth Defects Research Part A: Clinical and Molecular Teratology* 2003; 67(11):903–4.

120. Begley A, Coveney J. Wonder vitamin or mass medication? Media and academic representation of folate fortification as a policy problem in Australia and New Zealand. *Australian and New Zealand Journal of Public Health* 2010; 34(5):466–71.

121. Illich I. *Limits to medicine: medical nemesis: the expropriation of health.* Hammondsworth, New York: Penguin; 1977.

122. Scientific Advisory Committee on Nutrition. *Folate and disease prevention.* Norwich: The Stationery Office; 2006.

123. Scientific Advisory Committee on Nutrition. *Folic acid and colorectal cancer risk: Review of recommendation for mandatory folic acid fortification Summary.* Norwich: The Stationery Office; 2009.

124. Lawrence M, Chai W, Kara R, Rosenberg I, Scott J, Tedstone A. Examination of selected national policies towards mandatory folic acid fortification. *Nutrition Reviews* 2009; 67:S73–S8.

125. Rofail D, Colligs A, Abetz L, Lindemann M, Maguire L. Factors contributing to the success of folic acid public health campaigns. *Journal of Public Health (Oxford)* 2012; 34(1):90–9.

126. Al-Wassia H, Shah P. Folic acid supplementation for the prevention of neural tube defects: promotion and use. *Dovepress* 2010; 2010(2):105–16.

127. Taylor T, Farkouh R, Graham J, Colligs A, Lindemann M, Lynen R, *et al.* Potential reduction in neural tube defects associated with use of metafolin-fortified oral contraceptives in the United States. *American Journal of Obstetrics and Gynecology* 2011; 205(5):460.e1–8.

128. Rosenberg IH. Science-based micronutrient fortification: which nutrients, how much, and how to know? *American Journal of Nutrition* 2005; 82(2):279–80.

129. Crider K, Bailey L, Berry R. Folic acid food fortification—its history, effect, concerns, and future directions. *Nutrients* 2011; 3(3):370–84.

130. Mills JL, Conley MR. Periconceptional vitamin supplementation to prevent neural tube defects: how can we do it? *European Journal of Obstetrics, Gynecology, and Reproductive Biology* 1995; 61(1):49–55.

131. Holmes MV, Newcombe P, Hubacek JA, Sofat R, Ricketts SL, Cooper J, *et al.* Effect modification by population dietary folate on the association between MTHFR genotype, homocysteine, and stroke risk: a meta-analysis of genetic studies and randomised trials. *Lancet* 2011; 378(9791):584–94.

Case study 3: mandatory milk fortification with vitamin D

Vitamin D deficiency is the most common medical condition in the world (1).

Introduction

A conventional nutrition education axiom is that a person will receive all the nutrients they require in sufficient amounts so long as their diet follows three principles: variety, balance, and moderation. These three principles are at the core of advice provided in dietary guidelines and food selection guides. Yet, there is a nutrient exception. It is unrealistic to expect that sufficient vitamin D for optimal health can be obtained from most diets around the world. The primary source of vitamin D for the body is sunlight via the action of ultraviolet B (UVB) radiation on the skin.

In contemporary times, humans' lifestyles and living conditions have departed significantly from those that have existed for most of our evolutionary journey to date. People now spend more time indoors away from direct sunlight and for the first time in history the majority of people are living in urban environments so that when they do venture outside it is not uncommon for buildings and air pollution to filter out much UVB radiation. The effect of these lifestyles and living conditions is to reduce the primary source of vitamin D for many people. Yet, human physiology in relation to vitamin D requirement has not been able to adapt to these changed circumstances. Vitamin D deficiency is reported to be prevalent in many countries around the world (2) including those that have abundant sunlight (3). Vitamin D deficiency has been described as now being a 'pandemic' (4). Rickets, which occurs when the growing bone and cartilage fail to mineralize sufficiently, is the most recognized manifestation of vitamin D deficiency (5).

Mandatory fortification of food products with vitamin D to increase the intake of this nutrient is one potential policy solution to the vitamin D deficiency policy problem. In this investigation, mandatory milk fortification with vitamin D (MMFVD) has been selected as the case study for the food fortification rationale of adding a nutrient to a food to substitute for a reduction in exposure to the primary source of a nutrient (sunlight). Milk was selected as the food vehicle because it has been the most prominent vehicle for this purpose in the past, and is anticipated to continue as such into the future. In some countries the addition of vitamin D to margarine has been mandated but usually this is for reasons of achieving nutrient equivalence (Chapter 1) with butter and not as an explicit fortification intervention to compensate for a reduction in the primary source of vitamin D. MMFVD was selected as the representative case study of this food fortification rationale because it is the only case, i.e. it is the 'revelatory' case (6). Although few countries currently recommend MMFVD, this appears set to change as attention towards the apparent substantial prevalence of vitamin D deficiency around the world increases. In addition, evidence about vitamin D and a variety of health relationships is rapidly accumulating (7). In 2011 the US Institute of Medicine (IOM) released a controversial report on vitamin D reference intakes that is likely to influence future global MMFVD activities.

The purpose of the chapter is to present the findings of the investigation into the MMFVD case study. The chapter starts by outlining the case study's background. Then an assessment of the case study's public health benefits, risks, and ethical considerations relative to alternative policy options is presented. An analysis of how and why the 2011 IOM report on vitamin D reference intakes was made will be used to analyse policy-making for this case study as it is a likely portent of future MMFVD recommendations. A discussion of the assessment and analysis findings is provided. Emerging from the discussion are proposed future directions for preventing vitamin D deficiency. Finally the case study findings are generalised to construct lessons regarding the food fortification rationale that adding nutrients to food is evidence-informed and ethically justified in circumstances where there is a reduction in exposure to the primary source of a nutrient.

Background
Vitamin D and health

Vitamin D is a fat soluble vitamin that actually behaves more as a hormone than as a conventional nutrient in the human body. The term vitamin D refers to two prohormones: ergocalciferol (vitamin D2); and cholecalciferol (vitamin D3). Vitamin D2 is produced by ultraviolet irradiation of the plant steroid ergosterol. Vitamin D3 is produced in the skin following exposure to ultraviolet light that converts 7-dehydrocholesterol to cholecalciferol. Vitamin D2 and D3 are transported to the liver where they are metabolized to 25-hydroxyvitamin D (25(OH)D), the major circulating form. Further hydroxylation occurs in the kidney to form the biologically active 1,25-dihydroxyvitamin D (1,25(OH)2D) which binds to the vitamin D receptor (VDR) found on the nuclear membrane of cells of at least 38 human tissues and organs (8). The different forms have different biological activity, with the vitamin D3 form being approximately 87% more effective in raising and maintaining the circulating serum 25(OH)D form, and produces two to three times greater storage of vitamin D than does equimolar D2 (ergocalciferol) (9).

A number of years before vitamin D was identified and isolated, it was the unrecognized active ingredient in several interventions that successfully prevented and treated rickets. Rickets most commonly presents in infants and children and is characterized by weak bones, bowed legs and growth retardation. The adult equivalent of rickets is osteomalacia and is characterized by bone discomfort and aches and pains in joints. Both Mellanby and McCollum in separate experiments induced rickets in animals and then demonstrated the efficacy of cod liver oil as a cure (10) and a couple of years later it was observed that exposure to a mercury arc lamp or sunlight could cure infantile rickets (11). Subsequently, vitamin D was identified and demonstrated to be essential for healthy bone maintenance and growth. It serves this physiological function by promoting absorption of calcium and phosphate from the small intestine, extracellular calcium homeostasis, and mineralization of the skeleton (12).

The identification of VDR sites throughout the body has led to interest in investigating other possible physiological functions for vitamin D. An emerging evidence base, drawing on consistent findings from a number of observational studies, is indicating that vitamin D is associated with a variety of physiological systems and may have a role in mediating many health outcomes. In addition to its well-established relationships with the intestine and bone, vitamin D may generate biological responses in five physiological systems, namely, the immune, pancreas and metabolic homeostasis, heart and cardiovascular, muscle and brain, as well as controlling the disease process of cancer (8). The relationships between vitamin D and physiological systems, biological responses and vitamin D deficiency related diseases are represented in Figures 7.1 and 7.2.

Sources of vitamin D

Vitamin D originates from three sources:

1 Sunlight exposure: vitamin D3 is synthesized directly when human skin is exposed to sunlight. This is the main source of vitamin D for most people. Commercial tanning beds and solaria that emit 2–6% UVB radiation are also

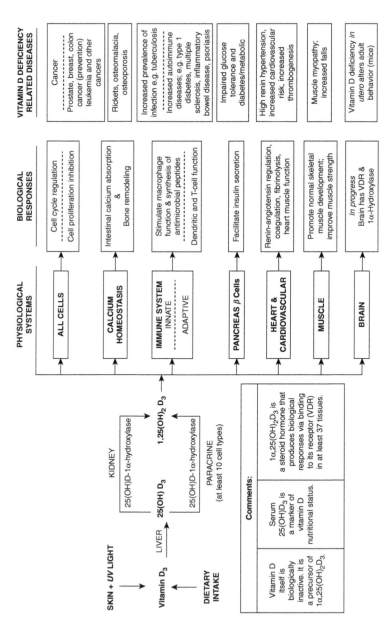

Fig. 7.1 Contribution of vitamin D to good health and diseases related to its deficiency.

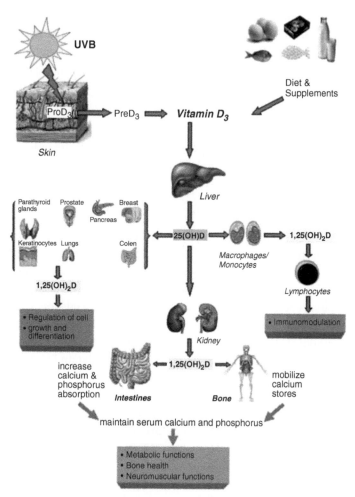

Fig. 7.2 Production, metabolism, and functions of vitamin D.

Reproduced with permission from the Sultan Qaboos University Medical Journal and the author.
Alshistawy MM. Vitamin D deficiency: This clandestine disease is veiled no more. *Sultan Qaboos University Medical Journal* 2012; 12:140–152. © Copyright 2012, Sultan Qaboos University Medical Journal, All Rights Reserved.

effective in mimicking sunlight in the synthesis of vitamin D3 in the skin (7), though as discussed later, they are associated with increased risk of early-onset melanoma and their prudent use is recommended by health authorities.

2 'Natural' food sources in the diet: small quantities of vitamin D3 occur in foods of animal origin with the richest sources being fish oils, flesh of fatty fish, eggs, and liver. Small quantities of vitamin D2 occur in some fungi especially if they are exposed to the sun.

3 Supplements and fortified foods: vitamins D2 and D3 are available from supplements and fortified foods (most commonly milk, margarine, fruit juices, bread, and breakfast cereals).

Recommended intake levels

It is broadly agreed that vitamin D levels in the body are best measured using the concentration of 25(OH)D in blood serum—it reflects the total 'intake' of vitamin D2 and D3 from sunlight and dietary sources. However, there is less agreement on what constitutes optimal, insufficient and deficient 25(OH)D concentrations because there are uncertainties about the quantity and quality of epidemiological evidence for a range of vitamin D and health relationships. Without an agreed cut-off level for optimal 25(OH)D concentration in blood serum, it is a challenge to set recommended vitamin D intake levels. As one reference point, the 2011 IOM Dietary Reference Intakes for Calcium and Vitamin D concluded that persons are at risk of vitamin D deficiency, inadequacy and sufficiency at serum 25(OH)D concentrations of <30 nmol/L (<12 ng/mL), 30–50 nmol/L (12–20 ng/mL) and ≥50 nmol/L (≥20 ng/mL) respectively, and serum concentrations >125 nmol/L (>50 ng/mL) are associated with potential adverse effects (13).

Among most European countries, a Recommended Dietary Allowance (RDA) which is the 'average daily dietary intake level that is sufficient to meet the nutrient requirements of nearly all (97.5%) healthy individuals in a particular life stage and gender group' (13) is used and ranges from 0–15 µg/day for adults in different population groups (14), where 15 µg equates to 600 International Units (IU) of vitamin D. In Australasia the reference values are an Adequate Intake (AI) (5–15 µg/day) which is used when there is insufficient evidence available to determine an RDA; in its place an AI is the 'average daily nutrient level based on observed or experimentally-determined approximations or estimates of nutrient intake by a group (or groups) of apparently healthy people that are assumed to be adequate' (15). Until recently an AI was the reference value approach in North America. Then with the release of the 2011 *IOM Dietary Reference Intakes for Calcium and Vitamin D*, a marked change occurred. Although an AI (10 µg/day) was still recommended for infants (0–12 months), an RDA of 15 µg/day was set for children, adolescents, and adults (including pregnant and lactating women) and an RDA of 20 µg/day for older adults (>70 years).

Vitamin D is a fat-soluble vitamin and has a potential for toxicity if it is chronically consumed at very high doses from fortified foods or dietary supplements. A Tolerable Upper Intake Level (UL) is defined as '[the] highest average daily nutrient intake level that is likely to pose no risk of adverse effects to almost all individuals in the general population' (13) and for adults has been set at 50 µg/day in Europe (16), 80 µg/day in Australasia (15), and 100 µg/day in North America (13). People with certain medical conditions including sarcoidosis, tuberculosis, lymphoma, and kidney stones should only take vitamin D-containing supplements under medical supervision. It is unlikely that sufficient naturally occurring vitamin D in food could be consumed to cause toxicity concerns.

Epidemiological evidence for the policy problem

It has been estimated that 1 billion people worldwide have vitamin D deficiency or insufficiency (7). However, it is difficult to estimate absolute vitamin D prevalence precisely as it will vary depending on what cut-off levels for serum vitamin D concentration are used to determine deficiency. What appears to be happening in some countries is that the prevalence is increasing (17). It has also been observed that in some countries where rickets was thought to have been eradicated it is now re-emerging (18).

Vitamin D deficiency is not spread evenly among or within populations. Population groups at high risk of vitamin D deficiency include (19):

- Infants who are exclusively breastfed: breastfeeding is the healthiest start for infants as it confers protection against infection and some chronic diseases, and contributes to improved cognitive development (20). Nevertheless, vitamin D is the exception to the nutrition guideline that breast milk is a complete food for infants as ordinarily it alone cannot meet requirements for this nutrient (21). The risk will be increased if the breastfeeding mother is herself vitamin D deficient.

- Older adults: aging is associated with decreased concentrations of 7-dehydrocholesterol, the precursor of vitamin D3 in the skin and therefore has a reduced capacity to make vitamin D3 in the skin (22). In addition older adults have reduced food intakes and so may have a corresponding reduced vitamin D intake but diet is not normally a factor in reduced vitamin D intakes, even in the elderly. They also tend to spend more time indoors, especially if they live in a nursing home or residential care. This is also the population group that is most at risk of falls and fractures.

- People with dark skin: greater amounts of the pigment melanin in the epidermal layer result in darker skin and melanin acts as a natural sunscreen reducing the skin's ability to produce vitamin D from sunlight (13). This presents challenges for dark-skinned populations moving from tropical areas with plenty of exposure to sunlight to more temperate climates e.g. Indian sub-continent populations migrating to the northern cities of England.

+ People with gastrointestinal disease: people with gastrointestinal disease often suffer from fat malabsorption—a condition that will interfere with the metabolism of fat-soluble vitamins such as vitamin D.

+ People who are obese or who have undergone gastric bypass surgery: because vitamin D is fat soluble, it is readily taken out of circulation by fat cells, a process that is more pronounced in people who are obese.

Cause of the policy problem

The primary cause of vitamin D deficiency is inadequate sunlight exposure. Dietary behaviour is not a significant contributing factor to vitamin D deficiency prevalence. With the exception of Inuit populations following traditional dietary practices characterized by high oily fish consumption (23), diet is a secondary source of vitamin D.

Although it is impossible to be certain about the lifestyles of human ancestors when they first evolved in central Africa, they were exposed to substantial amounts of sunlight and they wore few coverings. The vitamin D was synthesized through the action of UVB radiation on their skin although the melanin (responsible for dark skin pigmentation) tended to moderate this synthesis as it is highly efficient in absorbing UVB radiation. As people migrated from central Africa to regions of the world far from the equator, the strength of the available sunlight diminished in proportion to the latitude's distance from the equator. This phenomenon occurs because as the angle at which the sun reaches the earth lessens, progressively more UVB radiation is absorbed by the earth's atmosphere to the extent that, during wintertime in some countries, there may be little if any vitamin D3 synthesis (24, 25). Selective pressures on migrating peoples meant that adaptation to lighter skin colour was an advantage for survival as it enabled more efficient synthesis of vitamin D (26). The relationship between sunlight exposure and vitamin D status has been proposed as an explanation for the evolution of lighter skin colouration as an adaptive response to less sunlight for those humans who migrated from Africa to regions of the world far from the equator, such as the Scandinavian countries (27).

Now vitamin D deficiency is believed to be prevalent in populations living in countries with plentiful sunshine (28) as well as in populations that have adapted to less sunshine (29). In both situations a variety of lifestyle circumstances and living conditions have resulted in decreased sunlight exposure for large sections of the population. Various cultural, religious and social customs may require people to cover their bodies extensively by wearing clothing such as robes, head coverings and/or long-sleeved garments that have the effect of decreasing sunlight exposure. Extensive swaddling on infants is common in some cultures. Urbanization is a powerful predictor of low levels of vitamin D in populations around the world. It is associated with crowded cities, tall buildings, air pollution and people working in offices, all being characteristics mitigating sunlight exposure, as well as fresh air and physical activity more broadly. In addition, many people are unlikely to obtain adequate vitamin D from sunlight because their living conditions mean they spend inordinate periods of time indoors—UVB radiation does not penetrate glass, so exposure to sunshine indoors through a window does not produce vitamin D (30). These people include those who are housebound, hospitalized, institutionalized, employed as shift workers, as well as people with a disability and office workers who spend most of their daylight hours in front of a computer. Risks for vitamin D deficiency can be cumulative, e.g. an individual with dark skin who lives in a country far from the equator and who covers most of their body with clothing will be presented with multiple risk factors for vitamin D deficiency.

Challenges with translating the epidemiological evidence for the policy problem into a policy solution

It might be anticipated that increased sunlight exposure is the logical policy response to the epidemiological evidence for vitamin D deficiency. However there exist scientific uncertainties and complicating circumstances that challenge the likely effectiveness of a policy based solely on promoting increased sunlight exposure.

The major scientific uncertainties affecting the policy formation process are the:

- Dispute about the quality and quantity of the evidence for the range of potential vitamin D–health relationships.
- Lack of consensus on cut-off levels for serum 25(OH)D concentrations to determine deficiency, insufficiency, optimal, and excessive status.
- Lack of consensus on recommended vitamin D intake levels (in addition to the uncertain cut-off levels for determining vitamin D status, there is the challenge of having to account for the uncertain contribution of sunlight, variation with different skin colour, different sun exposure behaviours, and variation with geographical location).
- Difficulty in reliably measuring the vitamin D composition of certain foods (31).

The complicating circumstances affecting the policy formation process are twofold. First is the variety of lifestyle circumstances and living conditions that have resulted in decreased sunlight exposure for large sections of the population. These circumstances and conditions often are not immediately amenable to change and require investment to plan and provide options for increased sun exposure, e.g. identifying opportunities to include time periods for sun exposure within a daily routine such as walk during lunchtime when at work.

The second complicating circumstance is that there exists an opposing health message in relation to sunlight exposure. The UVB radiation that enables vitamin D to be synthesized in the skin also is a risk factor for skin cancer (malignant melanoma) (32). The use of tanning beds is also a risk factor for melanoma (33). In response many cancer prevention agencies have promoted messages encouraging people to avoid sun exposure, to cover up when outdoors and to apply sunscreen to block out UVB radiation. Some have suggested that such messages have contributed to vitamin D deficiency (5). Sunscreens with a sun protection factor of 15 or more when applied properly absorb 99% of the incident UVB radiation and will decrease the synthesis of vitamin D in the skin by a corresponding amount (34). Because people generally do not apply sufficient amounts or cover all exposed skin the significance of the role that sunscreen may play in reducing vitamin D synthesis is uncertain.

The challenge for public health agencies is to achieve a prudent balance with sun exposure advice so as to promote a sufficient vitamin D status for the population while protecting against risk of melanoma. Some believe that until recently the advice has been skewed too far towards avoidance to the denial of the health benefits to be gained from sun exposure. The argument has been made that in attempting to protect against skin cancer public health agencies have inadvertently created an environment of increased risk for a range of other cancers associated with vitamin D deficiency (35).

Assessing the public health benefits, risks, and ethical considerations of policy options

There are six policy options available to respond to the epidemiological evidence of vitamin D deficiency:

1 Mandatory milk fortification with vitamin D.
2 Voluntary milk fortification with vitamin D.
3 Public health measure—promote sunlight exposure.
4 Vitamin D supplementation.
5 Nutrition education.
6 Maintaining the status quo.

Each of these policy options is described and examined in terms of how they relate to the cause of the policy problem—vitamin D deficiency being a policy problem resulting from reduced sunlight exposure that is the primary source of vitamin D. The case for each policy option as a solution to NTDs is assessed in relation to its public health benefits (effectiveness, costeffectiveness, equity, and practical advantages), risks (primary and secondary and practical disadvantages), and ethical considerations—in terms of its adherence to five justificatory conditions (effectiveness, proportionality, necessity, least infringement, public justification). Table 7.1 summarizes the public health benefits, risks and ethical considerations of the six policy options.

The policy options are context dependent. In other words, the assessment of each policy option will vary depending on the local circumstances associated with vitamin D deficiency, including:

- The national vitamin D deficiency prevalence.
- The level of political commitment for the policy option.
- The latitude, season, and degree of urbanization.
- Whether other policy interventions will be introduced to complement a particular policy option.

Therefore, the assessment of each policy option is based on four assumptions. First, that vitamin D deficiency is prevalent in the local setting where the assessment is based; second, that the level of political commitment for each policy option is comparable with the current norms as reported in the scientific literature, i.e. not necessarily the ideal (this assumption is necessary because evidence is only available for current norms); third, that the latitude and season and degree of urbanization do not preclude the ability to obtain sufficient sunlight to achieve adequate vitamin D status; and fourth, that each policy option would be implemented as a stand-alone policy response.

Mandatory vitamin D fortification of milk

Description

MMFVD is not a common policy option, but based on practice in Canada, the original country that adopted this policy option, fluid milk is fortified to provide 44% of the recommended daily intake (of 400 IU or 10 μg) per 250-mL serving (36). Milk is a particularly suitable vehicle because vitamin D is fat soluble and milk is a good source of calcium consistent with bone health messages. However, it is not ideal for countries where the population does not drink milk, either because it is not customary or because they are lactose sensitive. For example, in India, bread might be a preferred food vehicle for vitamin D fortification (37).

Relationship of this policy option to the cause of the policy problem

MMFVD does not directly address the cause of the policy problem.

Public health benefits

Effectiveness In those countries where MMFVD has been implemented and evaluation has been undertaken, the results offer mixed support for the effectiveness of this policy intervention. Shortly after MMFVD was introduced in Canada in 1975 childhood rickets was virtually eliminated; however, cases of childhood rickets reappeared in the 1990s in association with the replacement of milk with plant-based beverages that were not fortified with vitamin D in children's diets (38). More recently it has been reported that in spite of MMFVD one-quarter of Canadians did not meet the vitamin D RDA (39). Similarly in Finland, MMFVD has been reported as having had a positive impact on the vitamin D status of young men, especially during winter, but one-third of this population group remained vitamin D insufficient (40).

These findings indicate that MMFVD is increasing vitamin D intakes in those countries where it is being implemented but not sufficiently for all populations groups to achieve recommended intakes or sufficient vitamin D status. Some researchers conclude that current levels of mandatory vitamin D fortification in permitted foods such as milk are likely to be inadequate to satisfy physiological requirements (41). Other researchers have commented that because milk consumption behaviours differ among population groups there is a need to not only consider increasing the amount of vitamin D added to milk but also increasing the range of foods eligible for fortification (36, 42). Vitamin D fortification interventions for a range of foods including those with a relatively low fat content (orange juice, wheat bread, skim milk powder) have been reported to increase serum 25(OH)D concentrations in community-dwelling adults (43).

Cost-effectiveness There is a lack of data available on the cost-effectiveness of MMFVD.

Equity MMFVD increases the intake of vitamin D for all people who consume milk. However, milk consumption patterns differ among populations.

Practical advantages MMFVD can deliver a dose of vitamin D to all people in the population who consume milk without the need for dietary behaviour change. Also it has the effect of reducing seasonal variation in vitamin D status.

Public health risks

The non-uniform milk consumption patterns among population groups means that there are practical challenges in designing a MMFVD intervention to achieve a Gaussian intake distribution for vitamin D with a narrow dispersion so that most people meet nutrient intake recommendations without exceeding the UL for this nutrient.

Ethical considerations

Effectiveness MMFVD has mixed effectiveness.

Proportionality Although there is potential to increase the vitamin D intake of relatively small segments of populations beyond the UL surveys indicate that, vitamin D deficiency is prevalent among populations. In addition, diseases with which it is associated, such as rickets, are severe. These circumstances support MMFVD as a proportional policy option.

Necessity Alternative policy options are available to help prevent vitamin D deficiency.

Least infringement MMFVD is the most coercive of the policy options available to prevent vitamin D deficiency. It has a high degree of infringement on an individual's free choice.

Public justification The degree to which people are made aware of the impact of MMFVD on their nutrient intake and have the opportunity to have the policy explained will vary among countries and with a range of circumstances.

Voluntary vitamin D fortification

Description

Whereas only a handful of countries have recommended MMFVD, voluntary vitamin D fortification is widely available in many countries. The food vehicles most commonly fortified with vitamin D on a voluntary basis are milk, yoghurt, cheese, fruit juices, and breakfast cereals.

Relationship of this policy option to the cause of the policy problem

Voluntary vitamin D fortification does not directly address the cause of the policy problem.

Public health benefits

The public health benefits for voluntary vitamin D fortification are similar to those for MMFVD with the distinction that a variety of food products will contain raised levels of vitamin D. Therefore, relative to MMFVD, voluntary vimtain D fortification is more likely to increase the spread of vitamin D exposure and hence dietary intakes across population groups.

Public health risks

The ability of voluntary vitamin D fortification to spread exposures and dietary intakes across population groups is both a public health benefit and a public health risk as people who consume large amounts of a variety of foods may be placed at risk of exceeding the vitamin D UL.

Practical disadvantages The design and implementation of the intervention— which foods are fortified, at what levels and when—are at the discretion of food manufacturers. Despite vitamin D deficiency apparently being prevalent in many populations, it cannot be assumed that food manufacturers would, or should, be responsible for controlling and treating this public health problem.

Ethical considerations

As for MMFVD, though voluntary vitamin D fortification is a less coercive policy option because an individual will likely be able to choose non-fortified food products.

Public health measure—promote sunlight exposure

Description

Modest sunlight exposure is being promoted by health authorities in a number of countries. In the UK modest sunlight exposure is described as an exposure of 10–15 minutes daily of sunshine (44). Elsewhere it has been estimated that exposure to arms and legs for five to 30 minutes in the middle of the day is adequate to meet vitamin D requirements, though this will vary with seasonality, latitude, clothing, sunscreen use, skin pigmentation and age, and some cultural practices (45). Modest sunlight exposure means avoiding baking or burning of the skin.

Relationship of this policy option to the cause of the policy problem

This policy option is directly related to the cause of the policy problem.

Public health benefits

Effectiveness In the absence of clear impact of vitamin D fortification and supplementation as well as an increased intake of vitamin D-rich foods, sunlight exposure has been demonstrably effective in providing sufficient vitamin D for positive health outcomes throughout human evolution. Similarly, it has been observed that during periods when sunlight has been less accessible such as the industrial revolution and modern urbanization, rickets has become prevalent.

Cost-effectiveness There is a lack of data available on the cost-effectiveness of sunlight exposure.

Equity Sunlight is free, and with the exception of those individuals who are housebound, hospitalized, or institutionalized, it is widely available to people. However, a person's geographical location (latitude and seasonality), culture and exposure to air pollution will affect the quality and quantity of the available sunlight.

Practical advantages Sunlight exposure is natural, and in addition to being effective in maintaining an adequate vitamin D status to prevent rickets, the behaviour itself is associated with broader health and well-being benefits because it takes place in fresh air and is generally accompanied by a level of physically activity.

Public health risks

Primary public health risk Sunlight exposure does not result in vitamin D toxicity even if undertaken for extended periods of time because its action is self-limiting with the sustained heat on the skin being thought to photo-degrade previtamin D3 and vitamin D3 as it is formed (7).

Secondary public health risk The UVB radiation present in sunlight is a risk factor for melanoma. Excessive sunlight exposure is the main cause of melanoma in most populations (46).

Practical disadvantages Sunlight exposure cannot reduce the seasonal variation in vitamin D status. However, Holick has estimated that sufficient sunlight exposure during summer, spring and autumn can provide for an adequate body fat reserve of vitamin D3 which can then be released during winter when vitamin D3 synthesis is less efficient (7).

Ethical considerations

Effectiveness Sunlight exposure is effective when accessible.

Proportionality Sunlight exposure is associated with public health benefits, but also public health risks when 'taken' in excessive amounts. It is a proportional policy option if modest sunlight exposure is practised. In Norway it has been estimated that the predicted increased cutaneous malignant melanoma deaths associated with raised sunlight exposure would be compensated 10-fold by the reduction in other cancer deaths from achieving elevated vitamin D status (47).

Necessity It is possible to prevent vitamin D deficiency without sunlight exposure if particular food selections are undertaken, including foods fortified with vitamin D, or vitamin D supplements are consumed. However, given sunlight's history of effectiveness, free availability and secondary health benefits it is an important component of a vitamin D deficiency prevention policy.

Least infringement Individuals are not obliged to be exposed to sunlight and as such this policy option has a minimal infringement on an individual's free choice.

Public justification Sunlight exposure is natural and is of benefit to everyone, its promotion is publicly justified.

Vitamin D supplementation

Description

Multivitamin supplements that contain 400 IU vitamin D3 and supplements containing vitamin D3 only in amounts ranging from 400–50,000 IU are now available (400 IU vitamin D3 = 10 µg vitamin D3 = 1 teaspoon of cod liver oil).

Relationship of this policy option to the cause of the policy problem

Vitamin D supplementation does not address the cause of the policy problem.

Public health benefits

Effectiveness Supplementation can be effective when implemented as a targeted policy option for high-risk population groups.

Cost-effectiveness A lack of evidence of cost-effectiveness.

Equity Not equitable.

Practical advantages Delivers a precise vitamin D dose to individuals without exposing everyone in the population to raised levels of this nutrient. It is particularly suitable for increasing the vitamin D intake of individuals in population groups at particular risk of vitamin D deficiency.

Public health risks

Primary risk Caution is indicated with vitamin D supplementation because vitamin D toxicity can be caused by excessive oral intake through too frequent and/or too high dosage of vitamin D supplements.

Practical disadvantages Requires an individual to be aware of the need to take a supplement and to comply with this behaviour. As a fat soluble vitamin, vitamin D can be taken monthly and still be effective (48). This will improve compliance relative to daily supplement usage recommended for other nutrient supplements because cost and respondent burden are lower.

Ethical considerations

Effectiveness Effective as a targeted policy option for high-risk population groups.

Proportionality As a targeted policy option, supplementation is a proportional policy option as the benefits it provides to high-risk population groups outweigh the small potential risk of excessive vitamin D intake.

Necessity Supplementation is not necessary, though in those circumstances where alternative policy options are not adequately increasing the dietary intake and status of this nutrient, it provides benefits, especially for high-risk groups.

Least infringement Supplementation is a low coercive policy option as individuals can choose whether or not to consume supplements.

Public justification Supplementation needs to be complemented with public education approaches to promote compliance and to inform targeted individuals about potential benefits and risks.

Nutrition education

Description

Nutrition education refers to the provision of programmes and materials designed to raise the public's awareness and skills in selecting, preparing and consuming a healthy diet containing adequate vitamin D in accordance with nutrient reference standards. In this instance, nutrition education is being interpreted to be exclusive of promoting prudent exposure to sunlight.

Relationship of this policy option to the cause of the policy problem

Nutrition education does not relate to the cause of the policy problem.

Public health benefits

With the exception of the traditional marine diet of Inuit populations, it is not possible to consume adequate vitamin D from a non-vitamin-D fortified diet. Nutrition education has the secondary benefit of raising the public's awareness and knowledge about vitamin D deficiency and rickets. From this perspective it is a complementary option to alternative policy options.

Public health risks

There are no public health risks.

Ethical considerations

Nutrition education is a proportional policy option in the sense that there are no substantive risks to negate the potential benefit that arises from informing the public of the policy problem, it has minimal infringement and it is publicly justified through its explicit action in informing people about rickets and vitamin D deficiency. However, it is unlikely to be effective as a stand-alone policy option and is only necessary as a complement to alternative policy options.

Maintaining the status quo

Description

Maintaining the status quo refers to deliberately deciding to not respond to epidemiological evidence of vitamin D deficiency. This policy option may be chosen to allow the policy maker more time to obtain additional evidence to inform an alternative policy response.

Relationship of this policy option to the cause of the policy problem

No relationship to the cause of the policy problem.

Public health benefits

There are no public health benefits of not responding to evidence of vitamin D deficiency because there will be no increase in vitamin D synthesis or availability in the food supply to prevent this policy problem.

Public health risks

There are no public health risks associated with a decision to maintain the status quo as there is no policy intervention.

When maintaining the status quo means choosing to discontinue a previously implemented policy option that had effectively prevented vitamin D deficiency, this policy problem may re-emerge.

Ethical considerations

Maintaining the status quo is the policy option which infringes the least on individuals and the population but it fails to meet the other four 'justificatory conditions' to support the case for this policy option—it is not effective, proportional, necessary or publicly justified. Given the estimated prevalence of vitamin D deficiency globally it is negligent to maintain the status quo pending the findings of long-term clinical trials (45).

Analysing the policy process: chronology of the making of MMFVD policy

A chronology of key milestones in the making of MMFVD as a policy solution to help prevent vitamin D deficiency and, in particular its manifestation as rickets, is outlined as follows.

1920s

Milk 'fortification' with vitamin D was being practised before vitamin D had been identified and synthesized. In the mid-1920s it was found that milk irradiation helped stimulate bone calcification in children because the irradiation

Table 7.1 Summary of public health benefits, risks, and ethical considerations of policy options available to respond to the epidemiological evidence for vitamin D deficiency

Policy option	Public health benefit	Public health risk	Ethical considerations
Mandatory vitamin D fortification of milk	Moderate effectiveness Moderately equitable Reduces seasonal variation in vitamin D status Does not require dietary behaviour change to increase vitamin D intake	Challenge to design MMFVD so that it delivers sufficient amount of vitamin D without increasing the vitamin D intake of certain groups beyond the UL	Proportional given the apparent high prevalence of vitamin D deficiency and severity of rickets. Not necessary if adequate investment in other, less coercive policy options
Voluntary vitamin D fortification of milk	Potential to spread vitamin D exposure and intakes efficiently across the population	The potential to spread vitamin D exposure and intakes efficiently across the population may result in individuals with high food intakes exceeding the vitamin D UL The food industry is responsible for implementation so difficult to control timing, level and extent of fortification	As for MMFVD though less coercive because maintains freedom of choice
Public health measures—promote sunlight exposure	High effectiveness in increasing vitamin D status and preventing rickets Equitable Associated with broader health and well-being benefits	Excessive sun exposure is the main risk factor for melanoma	High ethical justification as it meets all evaluative criteria, it is effective, proportional, has minimal infringement, necessary and publicly justified

(Continued)

Table 7.1 (continued) Summary of public health benefits, risks, and ethical considerations of policy options available to respond to the epidemiological evidence for vitamin D deficiency

Policy option	Public health benefit	Public health risk	Ethical considerations
Supplementation	Effective as a targeted policy option for high risk populations	Vitamin D toxicity if consumed in excessive amounts Practical disadvantage of requiring awareness and compliance to be effective	Ethically justified when used as a targeted policy option for high risk population groups
Nutrition education	Not effective in providing sufficient vitamin D for health	Nil	Ethically justified in the context of being a complement to other policy options as it can help raise the public's awareness and knowledge about vitamin D deficiency and rickets
Maintaining the status quo	Nil	Vitamin D deficiency and rickets may re-emerge if previously controlled	Not ethically justified as it is negligent to not respond to the substantial body of evidence regarding the prevalence of vitamin D deficiency and re-emergence of rickets

practise inadvertently converted inactive ergosterol into physiologically active vitamin D2 (49, 50).

1930s

In 1932, vitamin D was purified and isolated and shortly afterwards fluid milk in the US was required to have vitamin D added if the label declared it was fortified—in practice almost all milk sold in the US has been fortified with vitamin D since that time (49). Milk fortified with 100 IU vitamin D_2 per 8 ounces has been attributed as effectively eradicating rickets in the US and Europe during the 1930s (4). The involvement of the medical profession in promoting the benefits of milk during this period even led some to query whether milk was a medicine or a food (51).

Also in the 1930s, the US government provided recommendations to parents about the beneficial effect of sunlight exposure for the prevention of rickets (52) and in Europe it was government policy to promote fresh air and outdoor recreation and holidays (10).

1950s

Milk was in short supply at the end of the Second World War and into the 1950s and in a misguided attempt to extend the shelf-life of milk many local stores that sold milk added vitamin D to it if it was not purchased by the expiry date. This action led to a rise in the incidence of hypercalcaemia in infants in the 1950s and resulted in European governments prohibiting vitamin D fortification of dairy products (4).

1970s

In 1975, MVDF was introduced in Canada (39).

2000s

In the 2000s, researchers observed a re-emergence in the presentation of classical, nutritional rickets, particularly among dark-skinned, breastfed infants (5). Throughout the decade many epidemiological studies were published reporting evidence of a relationship between vitamin D status and a range of health outcomes.

During this period both Finland and Israel introduced MVDF (36).

2010s

In 2011, the US IOM released its report on Dietary reference Intakes for calcium and vitamin D (13). The vitamin D reference intakes are a significant change from the previous version of the document. Reference intakes that had been expressed as AIs are now expressed as RDAs and the values for most children and adults are triple those of the previous version while the UL for most children and all adults has doubled.

Discussion

The public health benefits, risks, and ethical considerations of MMFVD

In principle, MMFVD passively increases the vitamin D intake of the population and thereby helps to increase vitamin D status and prevent rickets. It is moderately equitable and does not require dietary behaviour change on the part of high risk groups or the population in general. There is a public health risk because differing milk consumption patterns present a challenge for policy-makers to set a fortification level that will help increase the population's vitamin D intake sufficiently without exceeding the UL for some groups. In terms of ethical justification, the apparent high prevalence of vitamin D deficiency and the severity of rickets support the proportionality of MMFVD though its necessity will diminish with adequate investment in other, less coercive policy options. In practice, in the few countries where it has been implemented, MMFVD is not achieving the level of health outcome improvement anticipated, though this most likely is a consequence of conservative fortification levels rather than an inherent flaw in the intervention.

The public health benefits, risks and ethical considerations vary among the policy options. The public health measure to promote sunlight exposure is the policy option that is associated with the greatest level of public health benefit and ethical justification of all policy options, including MMFVD. However its potential for promoting malignant melanoma if inappropriately 'consumed' requires caution in its implementation. Voluntary fortification broadly mimics MMFVD but at more moderate levels of public health benefit, risk and ethical justification. Vitamin D supplementation provides a public health benefit, risk and ethical consideration profile that is especially suited for a policy option targeted to individuals in high risk populations. Nutrition education has low public health benefits and risks though it is ethically justified as a complement to other policy options. Maintaining the status quo is not indicated as a viable policy option.

The assessment reveals that there is a relationship between the degree of public health benefits, risks and ethical considerations associated with each policy option and how closely it addresses the aetiological evidence for the underlying cause of vitamin D deficiency. The cause of vitamin D deficiency is inadequate sunlight exposure. The public health measure to promote sunlight exposure is the policy option that most directly addresses this cause. It increases sunlight exposure and in so doing increases vitamin D synthesis in the skin. An ancillary consideration is that many people living in modern urban environments would benefit from a lifestyle that incorporates increased exposure to fresh air and physical activity.

The alternative policy options to increased sunlight exposure do not address the underlying cause of the policy problem and have varying effectiveness in increasing vitamin D status. In addition, these alternative policy options are associated with a diversity of public health risks and adverse ethical considerations.

The policy process for MMFVD

Few countries have recommended MMFVD. In the absence of many examples for this case study, the IOM report on calcium and vitamin D Dietary Reference Intakes (13) was used as a proxy to analyse how and why MMFVD might be formulated. This report was selected because it is anticipated that it will be influential in shaping MMFVD debates into the future. This anticipation is based on North American Dietary Reference Intakes carrying substantial weight in influencing not just domestic food regulation policies but also reference standards and regulation policies in many countries around the world. This influence is a result of the capacity of the US and Canada to undertake high quality food and nutrition research to inform the development of such reference standards and the proportion of global food trade that originates and is managed by these countries.

Against the background of a growing body of evidence, the US and Canadian governments asked the IOM to assess the current data on health outcomes associated with calcium and vitamin D and to update the 1997 Dietary Reference Intakes for these nutrients. In undertaking this task the IOM work programme was informed primarily by two commissioned systematic reviews of scientific evidence (53, 54).

The report's recommendations included changing the AI values to RDAs, tripling the vitamin D reference intake for most children and adults (from 5 to 15 μg vitamin D/day) and doubling the UL for most children and all adults. The IOM committee based their recommendations on evidence of the relationship between vitamin D and bone health. They concluded that there was no convincing evidence from intervention trials of a causal role for vitamin D on health outcomes beyond bone health and as such potential additional physiological functions did not inform their recommendations. The committee also cautioned against the notion of 'more is better' in regard to vitamin D intake. Curiously, when preparing these recommendations the IOM committee assumed there was no contribution from sun exposure to vitamin D status. This assumption effectively meant that the potential influence of variables such as latitude, seasonality and skin colour on vitamin D status was not considered.

The report's recommendations proved to be controversial. In April 2011 the journal *Public Health Nutrition* published a series of invited letters critical of the IOM report, followed by rebuttal letters in the following issue of the journal, including one from the chair of the IOM committee (55). The criticisms ranged from concerns about procedural matters to the reference intake values themselves. A common criticism was that the report had failed to account for the accumulating evidence for potential vitamin D–health relationships. Critics were concerned that despite the values being set significantly higher than in the previous version of the recommendations, they were too conservative and not consistent with levels needed for optimal health.

This experience exposed the tensions and competing views when using evidence to inform nutrient reference standards which will in turn, have a bearing on food fortification policy-making. The debate centres on the question 'What counts as evidence?' when formulating policy recommendations. The answer to this question depends on how the relationship between vitamin D and health is framed and in particular the dichotomy between a holistic and a reductionist frame of reference (Chapter 2).

A holistic frame of reference conceptualizes the vitamin D–health relationship from the perspective that vitamin D status is a biomarker of a broad and complex relationship between sunlight exposure and health and 'well-being'. Because VDRs are spread throughout the tissues and organs of the body, it is likely that vitamin D derived from sunlight is associated with multiple health outcomes. The relationship between sunlight and health and well-being is the epitome of a holistic relationship. An anthropological perspective has been proposed to provide a method for estimating optimal vitamin D status. According to this perspective what would count as evidence for determining optimal vitamin D status for health is that measured in healthy people who spend most of their time outdoors wearing a modest amount of clothing and receiving sensible sunlight exposure (56). For example, it has been estimated that healthy men who completed a summer season of outdoor work had a mean serum 25(OH)D of 45 ng/mL (122 nmol/L), with some men exceeding 80 ng/mL (200 nmol/L) (57). By its nature this estimate would have high external validity but low internal validity in terms of controlling for potentially multiple confounding factors that affect relationship components such as measuring what is 'sensible' sunlight exposure and what is meant by well-being.

A reductionist frame of reference reduces the broad sunlight-health and well being relationship into a collection of single linear relationships. What counts as evidence in this approach is the evidence that is drawn from research methods that investigate the relationship between vitamin D status and individual physiological outcomes. Procedures for such investigations are well developed and represented by systems that appraise the quality of evidence by ranking the ability of the research method, for the study from which the evidence is derived, to control for bias and to demonstrate causality (Chapter 1). These procedures rank experimental studies such as RCTs, where an exposure is carefully controlled by the researcher, as providing high quality evidence. Observational studies, such as cohort and case-control studies, where the researcher observes and measures exposure, are ranked as providing lower quality evidence as they are unable to demonstrate causality and are vulnerable to bias. This approach provides evidence of high internal validity but low external validity—particularly as it does not capture the over-arching nature and scope of the relationship between sunlight and health.

The IOM report recommendations represent the outcomes of a reductionist approach to evidence-informed practice. It discounted evidence for vitamin D–health relationships that was derived from observational studies. Some researchers have commented that the evidence for such relationships is impressive but until clinical trials are conducted and causality and safety are established, it is premature to use the evidence from observational studies to inform nutrient reference standards (45, 58). These researchers highlighted previous problems with antioxidant vitamin supplements in which results from observational studies indicated an inverse association between several vitamins and the risk of cancer and cardiovascular disease. Evidence derived from RCTs subsequently showed they had no such effect and even increased mortality (59). The transferability of previous experiences of safety concerns is not relevant to sunlight exposure but is relevant to MMFVD.

From a policy implication perspective, the adoption of this reductionist approach has the effect of denying sunlight exposure as a policy option to address vitamin D deficiency. The approach was unable to account for the contribution of sunlight exposure to vitamin D status and health and its response essentially was to remove it from consideration. The resulting IOM recommendations, expressed as dietary intake amounts, predetermined that vitamin D be obtained only from dietary sources (natural diet, fortified foods, supplements) and not sunlight exposure. Some have suggested that the IOM's failure to countenance the contribution of sunlight to vitamin D status and health outcomes reflects a process driven by the need for the evidence to fit within the design of a reductionist orthodoxy at the expense of common sense (23).

Future directions for preventing vitamin D deficiency

Formulating a future policy for preventing vitamin D deficiency safely, effectively, and ethically is complex. Three priority activities are indicated: research; a two-stage policy response; and monitoring and evaluation.

Research

Ongoing research into food and health relationships is needed to help address the scientific uncertainties that are clouding understandings of this policy topic and the ability to formulate policy solutions. The research needs to encompass the full scope of potential sunlight and health relationships so that measures of excessive, optimal, insufficient and deficient vitamin D status can be better defined and vitamin D reference intake levels established.

A two-stage policy response

First stage Undertake a policy intervention to increase vitamin D intake for promoting bone health while ongoing research proceeds. The intervention would involve a combination of promoting sunlight exposure, supplementation, and nutrition education implemented in the following complementary manner to deliver increased levels of vitamin D to all population groups:

♦ Promotion of sunlight exposure: the promotion of sunlight exposure should be the foundation to the policy intervention. It directly addresses the cause of the policy problem and other policy options could then be built around it to target identified need in some population groups or individuals. This component of the intervention requires the promotion of sensible sunlight exposure while avoiding sun baking leading to sunburn and increased risk of melanoma. Sensible sunlight exposure means managing the time of sun exposure, the length of time exposed and what parts of the body are exposed (the face is particularly sensitive to excessive exposure).

♦ Supplementation: vitamin D-containing supplements are indicated for people in high-risk population groups and those who are housebound, hospitalized, institutionalized, as well as people with a disability, and where cultural norms involve extensive covering-up of the body, including infant swaddling. In addition supplementation may be indicated at critical life stages such as during pregnancy and lactation. There is an assay available to measure vitamin D status and this could be used as a screening tool for individuals within high risk population groups. Caution is required in interpreting the results of such tests as concerns have been raised regarding the assay's reliability (60). Nevertheless, in several high income countries it has become a frequently requested test. For example, in Australia, the number of people taking tests to measure their vitamin D status increased more than 50-fold between 2001–2011 so that in 2011 nearly 3 million tests were undertaken costing the Australian government almost $100 million (61).

◆ Nutrition education: obtaining sufficient vitamin D from natural food sources alone is unlikely for most people. Instead the purpose of nutrition education is to inform people about this policy topic and the policy options available.

Second stage Enacted if the findings emerging from the ongoing research indicate that increased vitamin D intakes across the population was required to achieve additional beneficial health outcomes. This stage would extend the first stage by introducing mandatory fortification of several commonly eaten foods with low doses of vitamin D to modestly increase dietary vitamin D intake evenly across the population while minimizing risk of excessive intake.

This two-stage policy intervention is intended to be a generic approach to thinking about policy options. It needs to be applied with flexibility because policy responses to evidence of vitamin D deficiency are context-dependent. Contexts such as a country's geographical location will have a bearing on the case for different policy options. For example, populations living in countries in Northern Europe generally have less access to sufficient sunlight to achieve vitamin D status recommendations than populations living in countries in Southern Europe. In this context the case for food fortification with vitamin D as a policy response to evidence of vitamin D deficiency is stronger in Northern Europe than in Southern Europe.

Monitoring and evaluation

Monitoring and evaluation will be an integral component of vitamin D deficiency prevention interventions into the future. Given the presence of VDRs in tissues throughout the body there is a high possibility that novel intakes of vitamin D will have a range of health impacts. Monitoring and evaluation activities will need to be sufficiently sensitive to detect the contributions of all dietary sources (natural foods, fortified foods and supplements), as well as sunlight, to total vitamin D intake.

Lessons from the case study findings for the food fortification rationale

Adding a nutrient to food to substitute for a reduction in exposure to the primary source of that nutrient was proposed as one of three rationales for mandatory food fortification (Chapter 1, Table 1.1). In this section the MMFVD case study findings are generalized to identify lessons regarding the plausibility of this particular food fortification rationale.

This rationale for food fortification is peculiar. It is the only one of the three rationales that is associated with one identified policy problem (vitamin D deficiency) and one underlying cause (lack of sunlight exposure). Therefore the case study findings provide direct lessons for the rationale's plausibility. Whereas the assessment findings indicate that promoting sunlight exposure is the best performed policy option to address the policy problem, MMFVD was assessed as having relatively modest public health benefits and risks and a modest ethical justification. However, modern lifestyles and living conditions militate against the likely effectiveness of promoting sunlight exposure in contemporary society. There may be no definitive policy option to respond to the policy problem. A pragmatic approach involving a combination of policy options is indicated (see 'Future directions', above). In these circumstances there is qualified support for MMFVD and consequently the plausibility of the food fortification rationale.

Conclusion

The MMFVD case study is unique in that it is the only example of using food fortification to substitute for a reduction in exposure to the primary source of a nutrient (sunlight). This situation arises because of the peculiarity that vitamin D's synthesis and its action in preventing rickets, along with stimulating a range of biological responses in many physiological systems throughout the body, is more typical of a hormone than that of a conventional nutrient. This peculiarity presented a valuable opportunity to assess and analyse unique characteristics of food fortification policy.

The principal lesson for food fortification policy-making that emerges from this case study is the profound influence of the framing of a public health policy problem on the shaping of the scope of the scientific inquiry and what counts as evidence. Currently, a reductionist approach is dominating the way that vitamin D deficiency is framed in the scientific literature and policy-making settings. Research inquiries are focused on investigating specific linear relationships between vitamin D and health outcomes. This approach is problematic in that lines of inquiry (at least those followed in the IOM report) are not only unable to account for the contribution of sunlight in explaining vitamin D-health relationships but they are actively excluding this factor. In this context it is not surprising that scientific uncertainties such as the determination of optimal vitamin D status persist. Consequently, there are challenges in precisely defining the policy problem and then formulating a policy solution.

A guiding principle for navigating such scientific uncertainties is to consider the causation of the policy problem. Vitamin D deficiency primarily is caused by a lack of sunlight exposure. The assessment undertaken in this investigation has shown that promoting sunlight exposure is the policy option associated with the best performance against public health benefits, risks and ethical considerations. However, the existence of two complicating circumstances (living conditions/lifestyle circumstances and an opposing health message that promotes the avoidance of sunlight exposure) presents challenges to the immediate effectiveness of this policy option. Currently, a simple and rational policy solution to the policy problem is not forthcoming. There are two particular policy dilemmas that are associated with MMFVD:

1 What quantity and quality of evidence is necessary to inform policy recommendations?

2 To what extent should policy recommendations be aspirational (promote sunlight exposure) and/or pragmatic (promote MMFVD and vitamin D supplements)?

In the immediate time frame, a staged policy response is suggested. Longer term there is much fertile territory for researchers to explore to better understand vitamin D deficiency and the potential 'sunlight–vitamin D–health' relationships. With the resulting rapidly accumulating evidence base, the nature and scope of this case study is likely to dramatically evolve. In the context of the current scientific uncertainties, the case study offers qualified support for the food fortification rationale of adding a nutrient to a food to substitute for a reduction in exposure to the primary source of a nutrient.

References

1. Holick M. *The vitamin D Solution: A three-step strategy to cure our most common health problem.* Carlton North: Scribe Publications; 2010.

2. Prentice A. Vitamin D deficiency: a global perspective. *Nutrition Reviews* 2008; 66:S153–S64.

3. Mithal A, Wahl DA, Bonjour JP, Burckhardt P, Dawson-Hughes B, Eisman JA, *et al.* Global vitamin D status and determinants of hypovitaminosis D. *Osteoporos International* 2009; 20(11):1807–20.

4. Holick M, Chen T. Vitamin D deficiency: a worldwide problem with health consequences. *American Journal of Clinical Nutrition* 2008; 87(4):1080S–6S.

5. Misra M, Pacaud D, Petryk A, Collett-Solberg P, Kappy M. Drug and Therapeutics Committee of the Lawson Wilkins Pediatric Endocrine Society. Vitamin D deficiency in children and its management: review of current knowledge and recommendations. *Pediatrics* 2008; 122(2):398–417.

6. Yin R. *Case study research: design and methods*, 4th ed. Thousand Oaks, CA: Sage Publications; 2009.

7. Holick M. Vitamin D deficiency. *New England Journal of Medicine* 2007; 357(3):266–81.

8. Norman A, Bouillon R. Vitamin D nutritional policy needs a vision for the future. *Experimental Biology and Medicine* 2010; 235(9):1034–45.

9. Heaney RP, Recker RR, Grote J, Horst RL, Armas LA. Vitamin D(3) is more potent than vitamin D(2) in humans. *Journal of Clinical Endocrinology and Metabolism* 2011; 96(3):E447–52.

10. Anon. Things may not be what they seem. [Editorial] *World Nutrition* 2011, 2(7): 308–32.

11. Hess A, Unger LJ. The cure of infantile rickets by sunlight. *Journal of the American Medical Association* 1921; 77:39–41.

12. Holick MF. McCollum Award Lecture, 1994: vitamin D—new horizons for the 21st century. *American Journal of Clinical Nutrition* 1994; 60(4):619–30.

13. Institute of Medicine of the National Academies. *Dietary Reference Intakes for Calcium and Vitamin D*. Washington DC: The National Academies Press; 2011.

14. Doets EL, de Wit LS, Dhonukshe-Rutten RA, Cavelaars AE, Raats MM, Timotijevic L, *et al*. Current micronutrient recommendations in Europe: towards understanding their differences and similarities. *European Journal of Nutrition* 2008; 47(Suppl 1):17–40.

15. National Health and Medical Research Council, Ministry of Health (NZ). 2006. *Nutrient reference values for Australia and New Zealand: Including recommended dietary intakes*. Canberra: Commonwealth of Australia; 2006.

16. Scientific Committee on Food. *Opinion of the Scientific Committee on Food on the Tolerable Upper Intake Level of vitamin D*. Brussels: European Commission; 2003.

17. Ganji V, Zhang X, Tangpricha V. Serum 25-hydroxyvitamin D concentrations and prevalence estimates of hypovitaminosis D in the U.S. population based on assay-adjusted data. *Journal of Nutrition* 2012; 142(3):498–507.

18. Nowson CA, Margerison C. Vitamin D intake and vitamin D status of Australians. *Medical Journal of Australia* 2002; 177(3):149–52.

19. National Institute of Health Office of Dietary Supplements. *Dietary Supplement Fact Sheet:Vitamin D*. 2011. [cited 22 April 2012]. Available from: http://ods.od.nih.gov/factsheets/VitaminD-HealthProfessional/.

20. National Health and Medical Research Council. *Draft infant feeding guidelines for health workers*. Canberra: NHMRC; 2011.

21. Picciano MF. Nutrient composition of human milk. *Pediatric Clinics of North America* 2001; 48(1):53–67.

22. Holick MF, Matsuoka LY, Wortsman J. Age, vitamin D, and solar ultraviolet. *Lancet* 1989; 2(8671):1104–5.

23. Gillie O. Blinded by science, pragmatism forgotten. *Public Health Nutrition* 2011; 14(04):566–7.

24. Webb AR, Kline L, Holick MF. Influence of season and latitude on the cutaneous synthesis of vitamin D3: exposure to winter sunlight in Boston and Edmonton will not promote vitamin D3 synthesis in human skin. *Journal of Clinical Endocrinology and Metabolism* 1988; 67(2):373–8.

25. Godar DE. UV doses worldwide. *Photochemisty and Photobiology* 2005; 81(4):736–49.

26. Clemens TL, Adams JS, Henderson SL, Holick MF. Increased skin pigment reduces the capacity of skin to synthesise vitamin D3. *Lancet* 1982; 1(8263):74–6.

27. Jablonski NG, Chaplin G. The evolution of human skin coloration. *Journal of Human Evolution* 2000; 39(1):57–106.

28. Khan AH, Iqbal R. Vitamin D deficiency in an ample sunlight country. *Journal of the College of Physicians and Surgeons – Pakistan* 2009; 19(5):267–8.

29. Tolppanen AM, Fraser A, Fraser WD, Lawlor DA. Risk factors for variation in 25-hydroxyvitamin D3 and D2 concentrations and vitamin D deficiency in children. *Journal of Clinical Endocrinology and Metabolism*; 97(4):1202–10.

30. Holick MF. Photobiology of vitamin D. In: Feldman D, Pike JW, Glorieux FH (eds). *Vitamin D*, 2nd ed, volume I. Burlington, MA: Elsevier; 2005.

31. Chen TC, Chimeh F, Lu Z, Mathieu J, Person KS, Zhang A, *et al.* Factors that influence the cutaneous synthesis and dietary sources of vitamin D. *Archives of Biochemistry and Biophysics* 2007; 460(2):213–7.

32. Wolpowitz D, Gilchrest BA. The vitamin D questions: how much do you need and how should you get it? *Journal of the American Academy of Dermatology* 2006; 54(2):301–17.

33. Beauty and the beast. *Lancet Oncology* 2009; 10(9):835.

34. Matsuoka LY, Ide L, Wortsman J, MacLaughlin JA, Holick MF. Sunscreens suppress cutaneous vitamin D3 synthesis. *Journal of Clinical Endocrinology and Metabolism* 1987; 64(6):1165–8.

35. Gillie O. Let the sun shine on you. [Commentary] *World Nutrition* 2011; 2(7): 308–32.

36. Calvo MS, Whiting SJ, Barton CN. Vitamin D fortification in the United States and Canada: current status and data needs. *American Journal of Clinical Nutrition* 2004; 80(6 Suppl):1710S–6S.

37. Babu US, Calvo MS. Modern India and the vitamin D dilemma: evidence for the need of a national food fortification program. *Molecular Nutrition and Food Research* 2010; 54(8):1134–47.

38. L'Abbe MR, Cockell KA, Lee NS. Micronutrient supplementation: when is best and why? *Proceedings of the Nutrition Society* 2003; 62(2):413–20.

39. Whiting SJ, Langlois KA, Vatanparast H, Greene-Finestone LS. The vitamin D status of Canadians relative to the 2011 Dietary Reference Intakes: an examination in children and adults with and without supplement use. *American Journal of Clinical Nutrition* 2011; 94(1):128–35.

40. Laaksi IT, Ruohola JP, Ylikomi TJ, Auvinen A, Haataja RI, Pihlajamaki HK, *et al.* Vitamin D fortification as public health policy: significant improvement in vitamin D status in young Finnish men. *European Journal of Clinical Nutrition* 2006; 60(8):1035–8.

41. Lehtonen-Veromaa M, Mottonen T, Leino A, Heinonen OJ, Rautava E, Viikari J. Prospective study on food fortification with vitamin D among adolescent females in Finland: minor effects. *British Journal of Nutrition* 2008; 100(2):418–23.

42. Vatanparast H, Calvo MS, Green TJ, Whiting SJ. Despite mandatory fortification of staple foods, vitamin D intakes of Canadian children and adults are inadequate. *The Journal of Steroid Biochemistry and Molecular Biology* 2010; 121(1–2):301–3.

43. Black, LJ, KM Seamans, KD Cashman, M Kiely. An updated systematic review and meta-analysis of the efficacy of vitamin D food fortification. *Journal of Nutrition* 2012; 142:1102–1108.

44. Ashwell M, Stone EM, Stolte H, Cashman KD, Macdonald H, Lanham-New S, *et al.* UK Food Standards Agency Workshop Report: an investigation of the relative contributions of diet and sunlight to vitamin D status. *British Journal of Nutrition* 2010; 104(4):603–11.

45. Lappe JM. The role of vitamin D in human health: a paradigm shift. *Journal of Evidence-Based Complementary & Alternative Medicine* 2011; 16(1):58–72.

46. Marks R. Epidemiology of melanoma. *Clinical and Experimental Dermatology* 2000; 25(6):459–63.

47. Moan J, Baturaite Z, Juzeniene A, Porojnicu A. Vitamin D, sun, sunbeds and health. *Public Health Nutrition* 2012; 15(4):711–15.

48. Ish-Shalom S, Segal E, Salganik T, Raz B, Bromberg IL, Vieth R. Comparison of daily, weekly, and monthly vitamin D3 in ethanol dosing protocols for two months in elderly hip fracture patients. *Journal of Clinical Endocrinology and Metabolism* 2008; 93(9):3430–5.

49. Bishai D, Nalubola R. The history of food fortification in the United States: its relevance for current fortification efforts in developing countries. *Economic Development and Cultural Change* 2002; 51(1):37–53.

50. Cowell S. Irradiation of milk for rickets in children. *British Medical Journal* 1935; 1:587–642.

51. Weart W. Milk: A food or a medicine. *New Republic* 1938; 93:359–61.

52. Holick MF. Resurrection of vitamin D deficiency and rickets. *Journal of Clinical Investigation* 2006; 116(8):2062–72.

53. Cranney A, Horsley T, O'Donnell S, Weiler HA, Puil L, Ooi DS, *et al. Effectiveness and safety of vitamin D in relation to bone health.* Evidence Report/Technology Assessment no. 158 (Prepared by the University of Ottawa Evidence-based Practice Center (UO-EPC) under Contract No. 290-02-0021). AHRQ Publication no. 07 E013. Rockville, MD: Agency for Healthcare Research and Quality; 2007.

54. Chung M, Balk EM, Brendel M, Ip S, Lau J, Lee J, *et al. Vitamin D and calcium: systematic review of health outcomes.* Evidence Report/Technology Assessment no. 183 (Prepared by Tufts Evidence-based Practice Center under Contract No. 290-2007-10055-I). AHRQ Publication no. 09-E015. Rockville, MD: Agency for Healthcare Research and Quality; 2009.

55. Ross AC. The 2011 report on dietary reference intakes for calcium and vitamin D. *Public Health Nutrition* 2011; 14(5):938–9.

56. Vieth R. Effects of vitamin D on bone and natural selection of skin colour: how much vitamin D nutrition are we talking about? In Agarwal SC, Stout SD (eds). *Bone loss and osteoporosis: an anthropological perspective.* New York: Kluwer Academic/Plenum Publishers; 2003, pp. 135–50.

57. Barger-Lux MJ, Heaney RP. Effects of above average summer sun exposure on serum 25-hydroxyvitamin D and calcium absorption. *Journal of Clinical Endocrinology and Metabolism* 2002; 87(11):4952–6.

58. Scragg R. Vitamin D and public health: an overview of recent research on common diseases and mortality in adulthood. *Public Health Nutrition* 2011; 14(9):1515–32.

59. Byers T. Anticancer vitamins du Jour—The ABCED's so far. *American Journal of Epidemiology* 2010; 172(1):1–3.

60. O'Donnell S, Cranney A, Horsley T, Weiler HA, Atkinson SA, Hanley DA, *et al.* Efficacy of food fortification on serum 25-hydroxyvitamin D concentrations: systematic review. *American Journal of Clinical Nutrition* 2008; 88(6):1528–34.

61. Robotham J. Experts at odds on vitamin D tests for pregnant women. *The Sydney Morning Herald* 2001: 3 August. [cited 18 May 2012]. Available from: http://www.smh. com.au/lifestyle/wellbeing/experts-at-odds-on-vitamin-d-tests-for-pregnant-women-20110802-1i9lp.html#ixzz1U8FQaE7R.

Section 3

Insights from the past and present, and a view to the future

This third section of this book provides the final step in this food fortification investigation. Its purpose is to present the combined research observations from the case studies to draw insights from the past and present practice of food fortification, and then to pose a view to the future of food fortification policy and practice.

Chapter 8 brings together the three sets of findings from the case studies presented in Section 2, and interprets and discusses them against the evidential, ethical, and political frameworks outlined in Section 1. This combining and interpreting helps build a coherent narrative about what has been observed regarding the relationship between the food fortification technology and policy objectives to protect and promote public health. This narrative provides answers to the investigation's two research questions in the form of descriptions of the public health benefits, risks, and ethical considerations of food fortification as well as the political dimension to how and why it is being made.

Chapter 9 presents a view to the future for food fortification. It discusses three of the more powerful drivers behind an anticipated increased food fortification presence in the food supply into the future: new agendas, new investments, and new technologies. The chapter then suggests priority activities for managing food fortification into the future as a technology for protecting and promoting public health.

Chapter 8

Insights for food fortification and public health

. . . there is an inextricable interrelationship between facts and values, both in the search for causes of disease and in the process of developing the best preventive policy. I argue . . . that their inevitable presence be revealed and their worth be publicly discussed (1).

(Reproduced from Sylvia Noble Tesh, Hidden Arguments: Political Ideology and Disease Prevention Policy, New Brunswick, N.J. and London, Rutgers University Press, Copyright © 1988.)

Introduction

This investigation began with the posing of two research questions about food fortification:

1 What are the public health benefits, risks, and ethical considerations associated with food fortification?

2 How and why are food fortification policies made?

The research approach to answer these questions involved breaking the broad scope of food fortification into the three plausible public health rationales for adding nutrients to food. This breaking down of the topic was necessary to help uncover the diversity of issues with which food fortification is involved. One representative case study for each of the three rationales was selected.

The assessment and analysis of each case study was presented in the previous section of this book. Each case study provided a distinct cluster of findings of the public health benefits, risks, and ethical considerations of using food fortification for a particular public health rationale, and the processes that help explain how and why it is being recommended in certain countries. Each cluster of findings was set against peculiar evidential, ethical, and political circumstances with which policy-makers and practitioners must contend when formulating, implementing, and evaluating food fortification interventions to promote and protect public health.

In this chapter, the findings from all three case studies are combined to provide a coherent assessment and analysis of mandatory food fortification. Combining the three clusters of findings enables patterns among the case studies to emerge, and provide more robust insights into the interplay of evidence, ethics, and politics in food fortification than might be obtained from a single case study. The chapter starts with a discussion of the answer to research question 1, followed by an overview of the implications that arise from this answer for informing food fortification policy and practice. An answer for research question 2 is then presented and is discussed in relation to its implications for food fortification policy and practice. Then, the chapter discusses the strengths and limitations of the research.

What are the public health benefits, risks, and ethical considerations associated with food fortification?

All mandatory food fortification case studies were associated with convincing epidemiological evidence for the nutrient–policy problem relationship under investigation. Yet, the assessment of mandatory food fortification as a policy solution for the different policy problems was associated with varying levels of public health benefits, risks, and ethical considerations. Similarly, alternative policy options to address the policy problems varied in their public health benefits, risks, and ethical considerations across the case studies. Here, the findings for each case study are combined and organized for their performance against the assessment criteria that were adopted for this investigation. The purpose of this activity is to help identify the existence of a pattern across the case studies to help explain the findings.

Performance against public health benefits criteria

Universal salt iodization (USI) was the mandatory food fortification case study that performed to the highest level against the criteria for public health benefits. This case study aligned closely with the underlying cause of the policy problem: micronutrient malnutrition caused by an inherent nutrient deficiency in the food supply. When micronutrient malnutrition is caused by poverty and food insecurity, mandatory food fortification performed less strongly against the public health benefits criteria. Mandatory flour fortification with folic acid (MFFFA) performed at a low–high level against the criteria, it did not align closely with the cause of the policy problem: neural tube defects (NTDs) caused primarily by genetic polymorphisms affecting nutrient metabolism in certain at-risk individuals. Mandatory milk fortification with vitamin D

(MMFVD) performed at a moderate level, it did not align closely with the cause of the policy problem: vitamin D deficiency caused by certain living conditions, social, religious, and cultural customs.

Among the alternative policy options available to tackle micronutrient malnutrition caused by an inherent nutrient deficiency in the food supply, none performed as well against the public health benefits criteria as USI, and none aligned with the underlying cause as closely as USI. Public health, social, and agricultural development measures are anticipated to perform better than mandatory food fortification when micronutrient malnutrition is caused by poverty and food insecurity. These measures are more aligned with this cause than mandatory food fortification. Among the alternative policy options available to tackle the policy problem of NTDs, folic acid supplementation performed to the highest level and approached, but did not exceed, the performance of MFFFA. It was the option most closely aligned with the cause of the policy problem. Among the alternative policy options available to tackle the policy problem of vitamin D deficiency, public health measures to promote sunlight exposure performed to the highest level and exceeded the performance of MMFVD. It was the option most closely aligned with the cause of the policy problem.

Performance against public health risks

All case studies were associated with a moderate level of public health risk (USI was low–moderate), although the prevalence of vitamin B12 deficiency and lingering concerns that it might promote the progression of colorectal cancer, mean that risks associated with MFFFA are potentially the most serious. A clear pattern linking the performances of the case studies against public health risks with their alignment with the cause of a policy problem was not immediately apparent. Among the alternative policy options available to tackle each policy problem, all were assessed as having a lower level of risk than the comparable mandatory food fortification policy option. The alternative policy option that most closely aligned with the cause of general micronutrient malnutrition, NTDs, or vitamin D deficiency, was consistently assessed as having the lowest or equal lowest public health risk among all available policy options.

Performance against ethical justification criteria

USI was assessed as having a strong ethical justification and it aligns closely with the cause of the policy problem it is addressing. When mandatory food fortification is used as a policy option to address micronutrient malnutrition caused by poverty and food insecurity, and with which it is not aligned, its ethical justification is weaker than that for USI. MFFFA was assessed as having a low ethical justification, it is not aligned with the cause of the policy problem.

MMFVD was assessed as being moderately ethically justified, it is not aligned with the cause of the policy problem.

Among the alternative policy options available to tackle micronutrient malnutrition caused by an inherent nutrient deficiency in the food supply, none had as strong an ethical justification as USI, and none aligned with the underlying cause as closely as USI. Public health, social, and agricultural development measures are anticipated to have a stronger ethical justification than mandatory food fortification when micronutrient malnutrition is caused by poverty and food insecurity. These measures are more aligned with this cause than mandatory food fortification. All alternative policy options to tackle NTDs (except, 'maintaining the status quo') were assessed as being more ethically justified than MFFFA, and folic acid supplementation, which is the option most closely aligned with the cause, was the most ethically justified. Public health measures promoting sunlight exposure were assessed as being the most ethically justified of all policy options available to tackle vitamin D deficiency, and is the option most closely aligned with the cause of this policy problem.

The insight that emerges

The insight that emerges from these case study findings is that generally the strongest predictor of high public health benefits, low public health risks, and ethical justification is the positive alignment of a policy option with the underlying cause of the policy problem. This is a valuable insight because it points to the important role of causation in providing guidance when considering potential policy solutions to address public health nutrition policy problems to optimize public health benefits and ethical justification and minimize public health risks.

The corollary of this insight is that caution is indicated when using food fortification for policy problems that are caused by social, religious, cultural, economic, environmental, or genetic circumstances. Food fortification alone cannot be expected to provide efficient or sustainable solutions for public health problems arising from these circumstances. Some have expressed frustration that using food fortification in such circumstances equates it to being a 'techno-fix' (2).

Implications of the case study findings for food fortification evaluative frameworks

Chapter 2 explained that protecting public health and safety is the primary objective of food regulatory systems when planning food fortification interventions. This objective takes on meaning in the context of evidential and ethical evaluative frameworks. The findings from the case study assessments

raise questions about many assumptions and procedures within these evaluative frameworks. They indicate that in their current form, there are limitations
for providing an evidence base that can fully and accurately inform policy-
makers about the public health benefits, risks, and ethical considerations of
mandatory food fortification (and alternative policy) interventions.
Implications from the case study findings for the four evaluative frameworks
that provide outputs to inform food fortification policy-makers are briefly
discussed.

Implications for evaluative frameworks for promoting public health

Public health and food regulatory authorities have invested in the establishment of frameworks that evaluate evidence of the ability of a food fortification
intervention to promote public health. These frameworks have rigorous procedures for guiding evidence retrieval, assessment, synthesis, and profiling
particularly through the application of the grading of recommendations,
assessment, development, and evaluation (GRADE) system, e.g. the WHO
evidence-informed guideline development process (Chapter 2). Typically,
these procedures have evolved from the evidence-based medicine movement,
and evidence obtained from experimental studies is highly ranked. This
approach is well-suited for evaluating precise linear relationships between
micronutrient interventions and specific health outcomes as evidence from
randomized controlled trials (RCTs) may be forthcoming. These relationships
were illustrated in the case studies in the instances of USI and reduced prevalence of goitre, MFFFA and folic acid supplementation and reduced risk of
NTDs, and vitamin D supplementation and reduced prevalence of rickets.

Conversely, the approach is less well suited to evaluating complex relationships between social, economic, and environmental interventions and multiple
potential health outcomes. Such relationships do not lend themselves to the
research design of RCTs, they are better evaluated using observational studies.
These relationships were illustrated in the case studies in the instances of sunlight exposure as an intervention to prevent vitamin D deficiency and possibly
promote other health outcomes, and poverty alleviation as an intervention to
tackle micronutrient malnutrition and promote social well-being. What this
means in food fortification practice is that when faced with evaluating the evidence available for different policy options, the design and procedures of the
evaluative frameworks tend to privilege micronutrient policy options over
alternative policy options.

The case study findings give thought to query the design and procedures of
the current dominant frameworks for evaluating policy options available to

promote public health outcomes. Is the observation that evaluative evidence for social, economic, and environmental interventions tends not to be rated highly by evaluative framework procedures a true shortcoming of the interventions, or is it more a shortcoming in the ability of the framework design and procedure to appropriately specify and measure the evidence from such interventions? The lesson from the case studies about the importance of considering causation to help guide the way that the relationship between a policy problem and a policy solution might be viewed as insightful to this situation. Greater accounting for causation of the policy problem is necessary in evaluative frameworks, because the procedure for determining what constitutes suitable evidence for informing a food fortification policy decision extends beyond rating the quality of evidence. It is also about taking into account the context for which the evidence is to be used (3). Being cognizant of the cause of a policy problem helps identify the nature and scope of the relationship that needs to be investigated, and therefore which type of research method should be used to evaluate a policy intervention.

Integrating causation into evaluative frameworks, at least to a greater extent than usually is practised, will require a reform of most frameworks' design and procedure. From a design perspective, assessing the cause of a policy problem needs to be confirmed as a necessary preliminary step in evaluative frameworks. WHO has recognized that this limitation exists with its guideline development process, and has indicated that activities are underway to attempt to remedy this situation (4). From a procedural perspective, the ranking of the quality of evidence needs to be reformed so that quality is assessed in relation to the context of the topic under investigation. In this regard, some are suggesting typologies rather than hierarchies as a way to better conceptualize the strengths and weaknesses of different methodological approaches (26). A typologies approach emphasizes the importance of matching research methods to the research question so that it is not just the quality but also the *relevance* of the research method that is critical in appraising evidence. By incorporating the concept of 'relevance of evidence' into appraisal approaches greater weighting in policy-making will be directed towards considering the appropriateness of a policy intervention in addressing the underlying cause of a policy problem.

A number of nutritionists are calling for such reforms to support an evidence-based nutrition movement to determine what constitutes evidence to inform policy and programmes in a nutrition context (5, 6). From an evidence-based nutrition perspective, what constitutes evidence to inform policy-making is the totality of the available evidence (7) or a so-called 'portfolio' approach which takes into account all types of relevant evidence in the process of informing policy and practice (8).

Implications for evaluative frameworks for evidence of cost-effectiveness

The evaluation of the cost-effectiveness of food fortification policy interventions is not a common practice. The challenges for these frameworks primarily relate to the assumptions and methods that are used in their planning and implementation and the interpretation of their findings. For example, the MFFFA case study demonstrated that the cost-effectiveness of different policy options in response to the folic acid–NTD evidence varies among research studies, depending on what assumptions were made regarding what costs and health outcomes were included/excluded in the studies. Critically, the ethical considerations associated with MFFFA are rarely included in the evaluation frameworks for evidence of this intervention's cost-effectiveness.

Greater investment in the evaluation of the cost-effectiveness of food fortification interventions is required to help inform policy-making processes. As part of this investment, the assumptions and methods of the evaluative frameworks need increased scrutiny and standardization. Inclusion of an assessment of the cause of policy problems as a preliminary step in such frameworks will help conceptualize the nature and scope of the relationship that needs to be investigated and hence help guide decisions about relevant assumptions and methods for studies.

Implications for evaluative frameworks for evidence of protecting public health

Risk analysis frameworks are used to evaluate evidence for protecting public health in the planning and implementation of public health policy interventions (Chapter 2). There is a conceptual and a technical challenge in using these frameworks for food fortification interventions. The conceptual challenge is that the frameworks are based on the premise that all risks associated with food fortification can be identified, assessed, managed, and communicated. The difficulty with this premise is that often food fortification interventions are novel, ie they have no history of use and in the case of MFFFA have been equated with intractable challenges (9). Inevitably, they are associated with scientific uncertainties, and the possibility of unforeseen risks arising from novel exposures to folic acid, iodine, or vitamin D cannot be discounted. Moreover, the case study assessments indicated that despite the significant ethical considerations associated with mandatory food fortification, these considerations were rarely if ever included in risk analysis activities.

The technical challenge for risk analysis frameworks relates to their historical roots as frameworks that were developed primarily within the discipline of toxicology for application to analyse toxicological risks. The frameworks have been adapted to a nutrition context by including a nutritional problem formulation stage and extending risk assessment to include both inadequate and excessive exposure to nutrients (Chapter 2). However, the uncertainty that arises relates to unknowns associated with the transferability of frameworks originally intended for toxicological applications to food fortification interventions. Nutrients behave differently to toxins, not least being that they are essential for health. It is not just relatively immediate safety concerns that need to be anticipated, but also frameworks need the capacity to analyse the longer-term and cumulative nature of nutrient risks, as well as possible dietary imbalances resulting from the food vehicles that carry the nutrients (10). For example, with USI the potential risks associated with excessive sodium intake on population blood pressure profiles resulting from the use of salt as a vehicle for iodine (this consideration is especially relevant to voluntary food fortification where often it is high sugar- and salt-containing foods that are the vehicles for the fortificant). This challenge is likely to increase into the future. The increasing number of food fortification interventions in the marketplace with overlapping micronutrient risks and benefits to analyse requires increasingly complex risk analysis approaches (11).

Faced with these conceptual and technical challenges, some have suggested an alternative approach to protect public health and safety in the context of food fortification—the application of the precautionary principle to decision-making processes. This principle seeks to avoid the creation of new problems while attempting to solve existing ones by anticipating unintended health consequences of public health interventions (12). A challenge with adopting the precautionary principle approach is that in the neoliberal political environment (Chapter 3) that currently frames food regulatory systems, it is likely to be viewed as stifling innovation. For both the conceptual and the technical challenges in using a risk analysis framework, the introduction of a preliminary step to conceptualize the cause of the policy problem being addressed by a food fortification intervention will enable key elements of the precautionary principle to be integrated into the risk analysis procedure. This will help place the risk analysis in context and more fully and accurately inform the identification, assessment, management, and communication of risks.

Implications for evaluative frameworks for ethical justification

The case studies have highlighted that mandating the addition of nutrients to food is an act with ethical implications. There were important effectiveness, proportionality, necessity, infringement, and public justification considerations associated with each case study and the strength of the argument for the ethical justification varied among the case studies. Yet, the ethical reasoning and moral values informing policy-making processes for food fortification interventions rarely are made explicit. Given the identification of scientific uncertainties with all the case studies, there is an added importance to include ethical reasoning in the evaluation of food fortification interventions. Ethical reasoning shares an iterative relationship with evidence-based practice with each complementing the other in policy-making processes (13). The inclusion of an assessment of the cause of a policy problem will help conceptualize the ethical justification of a policy intervention.

How and why are food fortification policies made?

The idealized notion of evidence-informed food fortification policy-making is one in which evidence is translated via rational processes to inform a policy outcome. The assessment of the evidence available for USI indicates that it is widely supported, and on balance it is associated with high public health benefit, low-moderate public health risk, and it is ethically justified. It is broadly consistent with a rational policy-making process. Conversely, in the instances of MFFFA and MMFVD, the assessment reveals that there are alternative policy options available that are associated overall with a higher public health benefit, lower public health risk, and higher ethical justification. An immediate explanation of the policy-making process for MFFFA and MMFVD is that both of these case studies are also associated with complicating circumstances that mitigate the likely effectiveness of non-food fortification policy options. For example, the proportion of unplanned pregnancies complicates the rational policy response of recommending folic acid supplements as a policy response to the epidemiological evidence for the NTD–folic acid relationship.

The adoption of MFFFA and MMFVD varies among countries around the world. Policy-makers are interpreting and responding to the public health benefits, risks, ethical considerations, and complicating factors in different ways. This variance in policy outcomes suggests that there are other factors at play, beyond complicating circumstances, which help explain how and why food fortification policies are, or are not, being made. In this section the findings from each case study, including the use of mandatory food fortification to address micronutrient malnutrition beyond iodine deficiency disorders (IDD), are combined to identify and discuss the interplay among actors, their activities, and agendas to help explain the food fortification policy process.

Actors

Each case study was associated with a range of actors with competing values, beliefs, and interests towards the available evidence for a policy problem and a policy response. USI to prevent IDD is the mandatory food fortification intervention that has received the highest consensus among actors as the recommended policy solution to a policy problem. This consensus is a key factor in explaining its wide adoption by countries around the world. However, micronutrient malnutrition more broadly is a policy problem that captures diverse views among actors towards the merits of mandatory food fortification as a policy solution. Many actors are now actively supporting low- and middle-income countries (LMICs) around the world to mandate the fortification of various foods, such as wheat flour and cooking oils, as a policy solution to micronutrient malnutrition. Examples of several prominent actors involved in such activities include:

- Helen Keller International has promoted private–public partnerships (PPPs) for wheat fortification with zinc, iron, and B-group vitamins, as well as oil fortification with vitamin A as part of its 'Fortify West Africa' programme (14).

- Micronutrient Initiative (MI) has supported the government of Nepal in issuing a decree that all flour processed at roller mills must contain iron, folic acid, and vitamin A (15).

- GAIN has provided financial support to the Ghanaian government for its national food fortification programme that involves fortifying vegetable oil with vitamin A, and wheat flour with vitamin A and B, iron, and folic acid (16).

However, other actors express concern that mandatory food fortification is a limited and potentially harmful policy response to micronutrient malnutrition in many countries. For example, in her review of the 'Fortify West Africa' programme, Sterken argues that mandatory food fortification interventions (17) are not addressing the social and agricultural causes of micronutrient malnutrition in these countries. She believes they threaten local food systems and existing food cultures as the population becomes reliant on technologies imported into the country. She also points out that those most at risk of micronutrient malnutrition are the same people least able to afford fortified foods, and questions whether public interests are being represented in decision-making processes. Others express concern that there has been a narrowing of the nutrition agenda through the international community's focus on micronutrients, at the expense of more fundamental food-based approaches (18). Food-based approaches are encouraged for helping deliver sustainable solutions to multiple nutrient deficiency problems (19, 20).

Actors have different resources and capacity to represent their views. The varying influence of different actors with competing interests is recognized in policy-making theory as an important determinant of policy processes and outcomes (21). For instance, powerful actors such as the Centers for Disease Control and Prevention (CDC), the Flour Fortification Initiative (FFI), GAIN, and MI have established strategic links with WHO, and have had access to critical policy activities. These activities include supporting meetings of the WHO's Nutrition Guidance Expert Advisory Group (NUGAG) and its sub-group dealing explicitly with micronutrients to update and develop new nutrition guidelines (22), co-authoring Cochrane systematic reviews, and contributing to WHO guideline development in general, as well as conducting strategic workshops and publishing reports (23) (Chapter 3). In the case of MFFFA, this powerful coalition of actors was particularly influential in shaping the policy-making process that resulted in WHO's 2009 recommendations on wheat and maize flour fortification (24).

These observations that there is differential capacity among actors to access policy-making processes are critical to helping explain evidence-informed practice in the policy process associated with mandatory food fortification case studies. As Marston and Watts comment (25): 'Being in a position to speak the "truth" can therefore be as important as what constitutes the truth'. This situation is common in the planning and implementing of policy interventions to tackle micronutrient malnutrition, where the people making policy decisions are not the same people who are experiencing the problems (26).

Activities

A variety of advocacy and framing activities were observed with each case study. The MFFFA case study in particular demonstrated the extensive and sophisticated advocacy of actors, such as the FFI, in promoting the adoption of flour fortification with folic acid around the world. FFI has a substantial amount of resources available to support people wanting to advance the case for MFFFA, and to support national governments in developing the relevant legislation for, and subsequent implementation of, this policy intervention. The ability of actors to visit individual countries and meet with key policy-makers has been decisive in the success of MFFFA advocacy. In the example of advocacy for MFFFA in Fiji, it was observed that this advocacy has been successful despite the lack of local evidence to inform this policy response. Some advocacy activities raise questions about the presence of 'white hat bias' in the policy process. White hat bias refers to the situation that arises when an actor pursues an action in the absence of evidence because they believe that the ends justify the means. They are convinced that they know the intervention will deliver the benefit and they have a moral right to undertake the implementation (27).

The framing of policy problems and policy options was prominent in all case studies. In the instance of USI, an important strategic action was to frame the policy problem as IDD, and not just goitre. With MFFFA, framing was frequently observed in the accentuation of the benefits of mandatory food fortification while diminishing its risks and ethical considerations. When the US Institute of Medicine (IOM) report on dietary reference intakes for calcium and vitamin D expressed its vitamin D recommendations as dietary intake amounts, it effectively framed the policy response as one that required vitamin D requirements to be met from dietary sources (natural diet, fortified foods, supplements) and not sunlight exposure. Some framing is subtle and may be unintentional, but nonetheless can have a decisive impact on what policy options are considered for a policy problem. For example, the WHO explains that a lack of essential nutrients in the diet characterizes malnutrition. Curiously, it includes folic acid as a particular nutrient of concern (28). Yet folic acid is a synthetic form of the vitamin folate, it is not found naturally in food. By framing the problem as a lack of synthetic folic acid, the WHO has inadvertently constrained the possible policy responses to this problem as being either folic acid supplementation or food fortified with folic acid.

Framing took many forms. It was exercised through the use of language, how benefits and risks were defined, and highlighting or obscuring the views of one group of actors over those of other actors. Framing was also observed in relation to what was not said or presented in policy debates. For example, ethical considerations associated with mandatory food fortification policy options were rarely identified or discussed.

Agendas

In Chapter 3, three particular agendas that influence the operation of food regulatory systems were described: dominant political ideology, global food trade and international obligations, and global health governance arrangements. The case study investigations focused primarily on global health governance arrangements, and the pursuit of PPPs in particular. This agenda has exerted a strong influence over the implementation of USI and its successful expansion to cover approximately two-thirds of countries around the world. Also, PPPs were observed to be prominent in micronutrient malnutrition activities more broadly, and in promoting the uptake of MFFFA in an increasing number of countries. The investigation into MMFVD with its focus on the IOM report did not explicitly analyse the influence of global health governance arrangements on this case study.

The case study observations lend support to the review presented in Chapter 3 about the influence of PPPs in affecting power relationships in the development and implementation of food fortification interventions. FFI and GAIN were observed to play a prominent role, not just in supporting the implementation of food fortification interventions, but also in actively shaping policy-making processes that led to food fortification recommendations such as those associated with MFFFA. It was commonly observed that among the variety of potential policy solutions to tackle a policy problem, the PPPs consistently expressed a preference for food fortification. By their nature many PPPs are designed to engage the private sector in helping provide market-based solutions and resources for policy problems. Food fortification is a particularly well-suited policy option for PPPs as it is a technology that can be developed, distributed, and marketed by food companies. Conversely, PPPs are often less inclined to seek out policy options that focus on the implementation of local food system interventions or social and economic development activities for poverty alleviation that can be especially relevant for addressing many micronutrient malnutrition problems.

Globally, PPPs are exerting a powerful influence over food fortification policy-making processes and policy outcomes. This influence is affecting the nutrient intakes and health of many populations. Yet, they operate outside of national government and United Nation (UN) systems, and as such are subject to less stringent transparency requirements in conducting their activities than if they were within those systems. In addition, the resources they have available to undertake public health interventions can exceed those of certain governments in LMICs. Given these situations, it is especially important that the accountability of PPPs be adequately addressed in global health governance arrangements. For example, through its business alliance network, GAIN works with companies including Coca-Cola, Cargill, Danone, Mars Inc, PepsiCo, Unilever, and Kraft, who manufacture a range of food products including some that contain high levels of sugar and/or salt.

The implementation of robust transparency and evaluation activities for the business alliance network will help alleviate concerns that in promoting food fortification interventions to address micronutrient malnutrition, GAIN might not also inadvertently promote the creation of a food environment that fosters dietary imbalances that contribute to diet-related non-communicable diseases. Philanthropic partners that fund PPPs also need consideration. It has been reported that the Bill and Melinda Gates Foundation will soon become the largest stakeholder of Coca-Cola and Kraft in the world (29) and faces similar challenges to GAIN in managing its food fortification policy and practice activities. The foundation has partnered with Coca-Cola in Uganda to increase production and distribution of mango and passion fruit juice (30), though there is no indication of juice fortification being a component of this partnership.

These situations highlight the need for good governance and safeguards within the UN system in managing global health governance arrangements with individual food manufacturers and other prospective partners including business interest non-government organizations (BINGOs) and public interest non-government organizations (PINGOs).

The insight that emerges

The case study observations illustrate that food fortification policy-making does not occur in a vacuum. The policy process for each case study was associated with a number of actors, activities, and agendas. Collectively, there is a broad pattern of interplay among these variables that helps explain how and why mandatory food fortification is, or is not, being adopted in certain countries.

It was frequently observed that there are competing views among actors regarding the evidence and ethics associated with micronutrient malnutrition, NTDs, and vitamin D deficiency and the role of food fortification as a possible policy solution to tackle these policy problems. Actors undertook activities to promote their respective views and the effectiveness of these activities depended largely on an actor's resources and capacity to have their views heard. In the instances of mandatory food fortification to address micronutrient malnutrition and MFFFA, the coming together of actors to form coalitions with shared views was instrumental in the success of securing these policy outcomes in certain countries. The ability of actors to undertake these activities and to have their views promoted or obscured was influenced by the underpinning agendas. For example, global health governance arrangements in the form of PPPs bolstered the capacity of certain actors to undertake advocacy activities and to gain access to important policy-making processes. PPPs were especially effective in giving voice to those actors promoting USI, mandatory food fortification to tackle micronutrient malnutrition more broadly, and MFFFA.

The insight that emerges from the case study analyses is that evidence and ethics do not speak for themselves in the policy process. Instead they are immersed in the inherently political nature of food fortification policy-making. What counts as evidence and ethics (and therefore what gets heard) is value-laden and varies among actors with competing views towards policy problems and solutions. For example, some actors may view it as unethical not to introduce MFFFA because it has been shown to reduce NTD birth prevalence substantially in many countries, whereas other actors may view it as unethical to introduce MFFFA because it is associated with potential risks and will increase the folic acid intake of everyone in the population who consumes the fortified foods. Whose view prevails and therefore what evidence and ethics is legitimized is predetermined to a large extent by underpinning agendas and the relative capacities of the actors engaged with the policy process.

Individually, the case studies displayed characteristics that were consistent with various aspects of the policy science frameworks reviewed in Chapter 2. The observation of the networking of actors involved with USI lends support to characteristics described by the network approach. USI is also associated with a strong evidence base, advocacy for expanding its coverage, and is represented on World Health Assembly policy agendas, illustrating how food fortification policy can happen when there is strategic coordination between the respective 'problem', 'policy', and 'political' policy-making components characterized by Kingdon's multiple streams theoretical approach. MFFFA displays characteristics consistent with the advocacy coalition framework. Globally, it is being assiduously promoted by a powerful coalition of actors who are engaged with a variety of sophisticated advocacy activities. Actors with alternative views are not engaged in coalitions of comparable strength.

Collectively, the case study observations illustrated that evidence was an important input to inform the food fortification policy process. However, as with the public health policy process in general, the way the evidence is framed, interpreted, and applied to policy-making is subject to prevailing values and political priorities (31). In this sense, it is itself an integral component of the political nature of mandatory food fortification policy-making. These observations are congruent with theory-informed policy science analyses of the use of evidence in the health policy process more broadly (32–34).

Implications of the case study findings for food fortification policy and practice

Chapter 3 outlined the inherently political nature of the food fortification policy process. In particular, it explained the critical roles of actors, their activities, and agendas in influencing policy-making. The findings from the case study analyses revealed the interplay between these variables in influencing the policy process. Implications from the case study findings for global health governance and implications of a deeper level of political activity for the scope of public health protection are briefly discussed.

Implications for global governance arrangements

Global health governance arrangements are having a profound impact on food fortification policy-making environment. In particular, the increasing presence of PPPs in the policy process is providing both opportunities and risks for food fortification activities. The case study observations highlight the need for further management procedures to maximize the opportunities and minimize the risks.

Prospective partners for PPPs such as food manufacturers, BINGOs, and PINGOs operate outside of conventional food fortification governance arrangements. Yet they are gaining significant influence in determining the nutrient composition of certain foods, the population's nutrient intake, and nutritional health. They have their own agendas, funding, and business models. For example, they are especially inclined to propose and implement market-based solutions for nutrition problems. This presents the challenge of needing to ensure that non-market solutions such as local agricultural programmes are not disadvantaged in the policy process. Certainly, food fortification offers an attractive technological solution to many nutrient inadequacy problems. With modern food processing and distribution systems in place it can rapidly increase a population's nutrient intake. However, in their desire to identify a convenient solution for a policy problem, are policy-makers undertaking a sufficient analysis of the circumstances and underlying causes associated with the problem? As Barker and Peeters comment:

> . . . a greater degree of influence over policy can be gained by those offering advice to government about solutions to problems than can be gained by those offering a deeper understanding of the problem itself . . . . It may be that governments ultimately are problem-solving organizations and anything that can be made available to assist them in finding solutions will be more valued than abstract understandings of cause and effect . . . . producing some solution – even an ineffective one which is, in fact, no solution – may be better, at least in the eyes of the public, than doing nothing at all (35).

Against this background there are implications about the legitimacy of decisions associated with global health governance arrangements and the need for these arrangements to be accountable. As Held and Koenig-Archibugi ask at the outset of their book on global governance and public accountability: 'To what extent are those who shape public policies accountable to those affected by their decisions?' (36).

The WHO has certain safeguards for working with PPPs (Chapter 3) but there remain calls for strengthening accountability in such arrangements (37) and the need to address what some have described as a 'governance gap' (38). In addition, traditionally safeguards have appropriately received a relatively high level of attention when UN agencies have worked with food manufacturers, but non-government organizations (NGOs) have tended to be less scrutinized. In recent times, it has been recognized that it is no longer sufficient to describe partnerships as being with NGOs, because NGOs is a broad term that might encompass NGOs representing business interests (BINGOs) or NGOs representing public interests (PINGOs). The case study observations indicate that this distinction is important but in making the distinction it is relevant to not overlook that PINGOs also exert their own values, beliefs, and interests over policy processes. Indeed, sometimes it can be difficult to distinguish between a BINGO and a PINGO and safeguards such as codes of conduct need to apply sufficiently across both types of organization.

Implications of a deeper level of political activity for the scope of public health protection

The findings from the case study analyses highlight that food fortification is a complex and controversial technology for protecting and promoting public health. They draw attention to two levels of politics that affect food fortification policy and practice. At one level of political activity food fortification is a technology to help protect and promote public health. At this level the political activity relates to the existence of competing views and activities among actors and the influence of underlying agendas, most prominently global health governance arrangements, which collectively shape food fortification processes and policy outcomes.

At a second, and deeper, level of political activity, food fortification is a conduit to profound changes in how food and health relationships are understood and how food systems are structured. At this level, the political activity relates to a degree of power and control over determinants of nutritional health. For example, promoting fortified wheat flour as a public health intervention in countries where wheat flour is not a traditional food can result in a transformation of local food systems and/or increased reliance on imported foods with subsequent social, economic, and political implications.

In the absence of a succinct definition of the food regulation objective, 'To protect public health and safety', too often risk analysis has been structured narrowly to focus on immediate safety concerns with less consideration of the broader public health impacts of food regulation activities (39). Earlier in this chapter, a suggestion was made to extend the scope of risk analysis to accommodate both the complex interactions of nutrient exposure changes resulting from multiple food fortification interventions, and the potential impact of food fortification on dietary imbalances. The deeper level of political analysis of food fortification highlights the need to further reform risk analysis frameworks. The framework's analysis should be extended to reflect a broader scope of how protecting public health is interpreted in a food fortification context. This means extending risk analysis beyond not only analysing changes in dietary intake (exposure) and potential health impacts, but also to encompass an analysis of the social, economic, and environmental impact of food fortification interventions on food systems.

Strengths and limitations of the research

Strengths

Originality

The research presented in this book is original and has been subject to peer review. It is especially strong for its novel policy science orientation. This orientation has enabled the research to provide evidence and understandings of food fortification as a technology to protect and promote public health. This orientation is distinct from the usual food fortification research focus that aims to provide evidence for an intervention to address a particular policy problem.

Conceptualization of food fortification

The conceptual framework that informed the research design provided a logic for organizing how to strategically investigate the complex nature of food fortification. The representative case studies that were selected within the research design are topical and capture especially rich evidential and ethical issues. Their assessment has provided an insight into the importance of drawing on the evidence of the underlying cause of a policy problem to inform the selection of a policy solution. This insight highlighted practical implications for the reform of the evaluative frameworks that provide the evidence and ethics to inform food fortification.

Critical analysis orientation

Critical analysis of mandatory food fortification is rare. This research included an analytical component to obtain an insight into the food fortification process in the context of scientific uncertainties, ethical dilemmas, and complicating circumstances associated with each case study. This analytical component was theoretically driven drawing on policy science frameworks. The insight into the nature of the interactions among actors, their activities, and agendas and the position of evidence within these interactions had practical implications for the food fortification policy process. Previously, when the policy process has been analysed it has tended to focus on voluntary food fortification and the tensions that arise from the competing objectives of public health actors and food manufacturers have been identified (2). Given mandatory food fortification is primarily motivated by public health objectives, it might be anticipated that there would be less tensions in its policy processes than those identified with voluntary food fortification. However, this research has demonstrated that policy processes for mandatory food fortification have their own tensions as a result of competing views towards public health policy problem–policy solution relationships among actors within the public health community.

Attention to objectivity and rigour

When undertaking policy analysis, researchers are irrevocably present in the design and implementation of the research as well as in the conclusions that are drawn. Their past experiences and moral views inevitably will shape the research process. Greater reflexivity (being aware of one's 'voice' and 'position' in research) on the part of researchers through an analysis of their involvement in defining research agendas and generating knowledge contributes to the strength of health policy analysis (40). The strength of this present food fortification research is illustrated through the procedures that were instigated to identify and manage this researcher's voice and position in the research.

From the outset (see the book's preface) the reader's attention was drawn to the author's presence in the research. This researcher attempted to adopt a stance of objectivity and neutrality with regard to the design, conduct, and interpretation of the research through the application of two particular actions. First, a conceptual framework was developed and applied to explicitly outline the logic that informed how the investigation was structured and the specific case studies were selected so as to each represent one of three plausible rationales for food fortification. Second, when assessing and analysing the case studies, this researcher attempted to provide a balanced account by presenting all major views on a topic. In addition, particular attention was directed towards highlighting the scientific uncertainties, ethical dilemmas, and presence of complicating factors with each case study. In this way the reader was made aware of the complexity of the case studies. The purpose of this action was to encourage the reader not to think of case studies as being definitively good or bad policies, but to gain a deeper understanding of the reasoning behind the views and actions of all prominent actors involved with the case study.

Limitations

Food fortification is a broad and complex research topic. Necessarily certain parameters needed to be put in place and assumptions made so that the research could be managed efficiently. These actions meant that the following limitations with the research could not be avoided.

Parameters placed on the selection of case studies and plausible rationales for food fortification

The parameters adopted in this research confined the investigation to select one case study for each of three rationales for mandatory food fortification. Each case study was selected to be representative of a policy problem linked to one food fortification rationale. Nevertheless, in the future this research approach would benefit from the inclusion of case studies to investigate different policy problem–problem causation relationships. For example, an investigation of food fortification to address the policy problem of micronutrient malnutrition when the cause was not an inherent nutrient deficiency in the food supply was addressed in a secondary manner only and within the USI case study. A case study investigation for the policy problem of micronutrient malnutrition when the cause is a parasite infection or related medical condition was not included in the research.

It was judged that at the current point in time the three rationales captured all possible circumstances for food fortification. In the future this may not be the case as other circumstances might arise. Changing environmental circumstances may create new rationales for food fortification. For instance, in the context that concerns about the contribution of greenhouse gas emissions to climate change may promote a reduction in red meat and milk consumption, some have suggested food fortification with iron and calcium may be required (41). From the other side of the food–environment relationship, other rationales for introducing food fortification may emerge. Environmental changes such as climate change, soil degradation, and water availability may influence the yield (42) and macronutrient composition (43) of certain crops, and indirectly reduce a population's micronutrient intake by lowering the quality of micronutrient-rich perishable foods (44).

Assumptions associated with the assessment of the case studies

The policy options available to address a policy problem are context-dependent. This means that their performance against assessment criteria may vary depending on local circumstances such as the prevalence of the policy problem, the level of political commitment, and resources invested in the implementation of the policy option, and whether other policy interventions will be available to complement the policy option. It was not realistic to assess each policy option under all contextual variations. Instead standard assumptions for each policy option in each case study were applied to the assessment process. These standard assumptions included that the policy problem was prevalent, that the level of political commitment to the option was modest, and that each policy option was implemented as a stand-alone option.

In practice, the assumptions might not be accurate and the performance of a policy option may vary from that reported in the research assessment if different circumstances were at play. For example, as a policy option to tackle micronutrient malnutrition, it is usually recommended that food fortification be implemented not as a stand-alone policy option but strategically as part of a broad based programme involving complementary policy options (45). Implemented in this way, its performance against the assessment criteria may vary to that reported. In relation to policy options such as promoting supplementation or public health measures, a greater political commitment to their implementation than currently occurs in most countries would likely result in a significant increase in their effectiveness beyond that reported.

Assumptions associated with the analysis of the case studies

The policy process associated with each case study is multifaceted. Necessarily, this research made several assumptions in capturing the scope and detail of each case study's policy process so that the data were sufficient to conduct the analyses. In relation to scope, the assumption was made that analysing case studies primarily from an international perspective would provide a plausible explanation of how and why each case study was being made. Information available for processes at national levels was included, but overall the analysis focused on international actors, advocacy, and framing activities at the international level and the global health governance agenda. The research was limited in its ability to capture national level actors and their activities and the influence on national conditions of neoliberal ideology and global food trade agendas.

In relation to detail the assumption was made that setting out a chronology organized around the primary milestones, actors, activities, and agendas in the case study's history was sufficient to make sense of how and why each case study was made. It was further assumed that sufficient data to prepare this chronology were available in food fortification policy-related documents such as scientific publications and official documentation available in the public domain. Therefore the research was limited in its ability to analyse intricate details of each case study and it was unable to collect data that might only be available from non-documentary sources.

References

1. Tesh SN. *Hidden arguments: political ideology and disease prevention policy.* New Brunswick, NJ: Rutgers University Press; 1988.
2. Nestle M. *Food politics: how the food industry influences nutrition and health.* Berkley, CA: University of California Press; 2002.
3. Dobrow M, Goel V, Upshur R. Evidence-based health policy: context and utilisation. *Social Science and Medicine* 2004; 58(1):207–17.
4. Pena-Rosas J, De-Regil L, Rogers L, Bopardikar A, Panisset U. Translating research into action: WHO evidence-informed guidelines for safe and effective micronutrient interventions. *Journal of Nutrition* 2012; 142(1):197S–204S.
5. Margetts B, Warm D, Yngve A, Sjostrom M. Developing an evidence-based approach to public health nutrition: translating evidence into policy. *Public Health Nutrition* 2001; 4(6A):1393–7.

6. Truswell AS. Levels and kinds of evidence for public-health nutrition. *Lancet* 2001; 357(9262):1061–2.

7. Kraemer K, de Pee S, Badham J. Evidence in multiple micronutrient nutrition: from history to science to effective programs. *Journal of Nutrition* 2012; 142(1):138S–42S.

8. James WPT. *Rio2012*. What next. Coming to judgement [Commentary]. *World Nutrition* 2012; 3(5):179–202 [cited 26 August 2012]. Available from: http://www. wphna.org.

9. Lawrence, M. Challenges in translating scientific evidence into mandatory food fortification policy: an antipodean case study of the folate-neural tube defect relationship. *Public Health Nutrition* 2005; 8(8):1235–41.

10. Meltzer HM, Aro A, Andersen NL, Koch B, Alexander J. Risk analysis applied to food fortification. *Public Health Nutrition* 2003; 6(3):281–91.

11. Verkerk RH. The paradox of overlapping micronutrient risks and benefits obligates risk/benefit analysis. *Toxicology* 2010; 278(1):27–38.

12. Kriebel D, Tickner J. Reenergizing public health through precaution. *American Journal of Public Health* 2001; 91(9):1351–5.

13. Carter S, Rychetnik L, Lloyd B, Kerridge I, Baur L, Bauman A, *et al.* Evidence, ethics, and values: a framework for health promotion. *American Journal of Public Health* 2011; 101(3):465–72.

14. Sablah M, Klopp J, Steinberg D, Baker S. Private-public partnerships drive one solution to vitamin and mineral deficiencies: 'Fortify West Africa'. *SCN News Nutrition and Business: How to Engage?* 2011; 39:40–4.

15. Micronutrient Initiative. *Micronutrient Initiative supports mandatory flour fortification in Nepal to improve health of the most vulnerable*, 2011 [cited 9 October 2012]. Available from: http://www.micronutrient.org/English/view.asp?x=656&id=49.

16. Global Alliance for Improved Nutrition. *Ghana launches national food fortification program*. Accra: GAIN; 3 October 2007 [Press release]. [cited 2 August, 2011]. Available from: http://www.gainhealth.org/press-releases/ghana-launches-national-food-fortification-program.

17. Sterken E. *Private-public partnerships drive one solution to vitamin and mineral deficiencies: 'Fortify West Africa'—A review*; 2012.

18. Pelletier DL, Menon P, Ngo T, Frongillo EA, Frongillo D. The nutrition policy process: the role of strategic capacity in advancing national nutrition agendas. *Food and Nutrition Bulletin* 2011; 32(2 Suppl):S59–69.

19. Blasbalg TL, Wispelwey B, Deckelbaum RJ. Econutrition and utilization of food-based approaches for nutritional health. *Food and Nutrition Bulletin* 201132(1 Suppl):S4–13.

20. Food and Agriculture Organization. *International Scientific Symposium on Biodiversity and Sustainable Diet: United against hunger.* FAO: Rome; November 2010.

21. Buse K, Mays, N, Walt, G. *Making health policy*. Maidenhead: Open University Press; 2005.

22. World Health Organization. *First Meeting of the WHO Nutrition Guidance Expert Advisory Group (NUGAG): Subgroups on Micronutrients, and Diet and Health*. [cited 11 October 2011]. Available from: http://www.who.int/nutrition/topics/NUGAG_meeting/en/index.html.

23. Serdula M, Peña-Rosas JP, Maberly GF, Parvanta I (eds). Flour fortification with iron, folic acid, vitamin B12, vitamin A, and zinc: Proceedings of the Second Technical Workshop on Wheat Flour Fortification. *Food and Nutrition Bulletin* 2010; 31(Suppl 1). [cited 13 May 2012]. Available from: http://nsinf.publisher.ingentaconnect.com/content/nsinf/fnb; jsessionid=hcpdc577vs2n.alice.

24. World Health Organization. *Recommendations on wheat and maize flour fortification meeting report: interim consensus statement.* 2009 [cited 28 March 2012]. Available from: http://www.who.int/nutrition/publications/micronutrients/wheat_maize_fortification/en/index.html.

25. Marston G, Watts, R. Tampering with the evidence: a critical appraisal of evidence-based policy-making. *The drawing board: An Australia review of public affairs.* 2003; 3(3):143–63.

26. Schuftan C. *Let us hope that the SUN initiative can really put nutrition at the centre of development.* [Column]. Website of the World Public Health Nutrition Association, January 2012. [cited 9 October 2012]. Available from: http://www.wphna.org.

27. Cope MB, Allison DB. White hat bias: examples of its presence in obesity research and a call for renewed commitment to faithfulness in research reporting. *International Journal of Obesity (Lond)* 2010; 34(1):84–8; discussion 3.

28. World Health Organization. *Nutrition: The department.* [cited 27 March 2012]. Available from: http://www.who.int/nutrition/about_us/en/.

29. Stuckler D, Basu S, McKee M. Global health philanthropy and institutional relationships: how should conflicts of interest be addressed? *PLoS Medicine* 2011; 8(4):e1001020.

30. Kasozi J. *Uganda: fruit farmers to reap from Coca-Cola, Gates Project.* [cited 1 May 2012]. Available from: http://allafrica.com/stories/201003030136.html.

31. Rychetnik L, Hawe P, Waters E, Barratt A, Frommer M. A glossary for evidence based public health. *Journal of Epidemiology and Community Health* 2004; 58(7):538–45.

32. Jewell CJ, Bero LA. 'Developing good taste in evidence': facilitators of and hindrances to evidence-informed health policymaking in state government. *Milbank Quarterly* 2008; 86(2):177–208.

33. Robeson P, Dobbins M, DeCorby K, Tirilis D. Facilitating access to pre-processed research evidence in public health. *BMC Public Health* 2010; 10:95.

34. Bowen S, Erickson T, Martens PJ, Crockett S. More than 'using research': the real challenges in promoting evidence-informed decision-making. *Healthcare Policy* 2009; 4(3):87–102.

35. Peters GB, Barker A. *Introduction: governments, information, advice and policy-making. Advising West European governments: inquiries, expertise and public policy.* Edinburgh: Edinburgh University Press; 1993.

36. Held D, Koenig-Archibugi, M (eds). *Global governance and public accountability.* Oxford: Blackwell Publishing; 2005.

37. Kraak V, Swinburn, B, Lawrence, M, Harrison, P. The accountability of public–private partnerships with food, beverage and restaurant companies to address global hunger and the double burden of malnutrition. *SCN News. Nutrition and Business: How to Engage?* 2011; 39, 11–24 [cited 3 June 2012]. Available from: http://www.unscn.org/files/Publications/SCN_News/SCNNEWS39_10.01_high_def.pdf.

38. Hawkes C, Buse, K. Public-private engagement for diet and health: addressing the governance gap. *SCN News Nutrition and Business: How to Engage?* 2011; 39:6–10.

39. Lawrence M. Do food regulatory systems protect public health? [Invited commentary] *Public Health Nutrition* 2009; 12(11):2247–9.

40. Walt G, Shiffman, J, Schneider, H, Murray, SF, Brugha, R & Gilson, L. 'Doing' health policy analysis: methodological and conceptual reflections and challenges. *Health Policy and Planning* 2008; 23(5):308–17.

41. Millward DJ, Garnett T. Plenary Lecture 3: Food and the planet: nutritional dilemmas of greenhouse gas emission reductions through reduced intakes of meat and dairy foods. *Proceedings of the Nutrition Society* 2009; 69(1):103–18.

42. Lobell DB, Schlenker W, Costa-Roberts J. Climate trends and global crop production since 1980. *Science* 2011; 333(6042):616–20.

43. Bloom AJ, Burger M, Rubio Asensio JS, Cousins AB. Carbon dioxide enrichment inhibits nitrate assimilation in wheat and Arabidopsis. *Science* 2010; 328(5980):899–903.

44. Edwards F, Dixon J, Friel S, Hall G, Hannigan I, Hattersley L, Hogan A, Larsen K, Lawrence M, Lockie S, Lopata A, Wilson R, Wood, B. *Food Systems, Climate Change Adaptation and Human Health in Australia.* State of the Science and Policy Discussion Paper Series. Canberra: National Climate Change Adaptation Research Facility: Adaptation Research Network—Human Health; 2011.

45. Allen L, de Benoist B, Dary O, Hurrell R. *Guidelines on food fortification with micronutrients.* Geneva: World Health Organization; 2006 [cited 8 October 2012]. Available from: http://www.who.int/nutrition/publications/guide_food_fortification_micronutrients.pdf.

Chapter 9

A view to the future

Our [Flour Fortification Initiative] aspirational goal is for 80% of the world's wheat flour from industrial mills to be fortified by 2015 (1).

GAIN's goal is to reach 1.5 billion people with fortified foods that have sustainable nutritional impact (2).

Introduction

It is almost 100 years since a confluence of nutrition knowledge and food science skills resulted in food fortification being developed as a technology to help prevent a public health problem (goitre). In the intervening years, a diversity of mandatory food fortification interventions has been implemented in countries around the world for the purpose of protecting and promoting public health. There has been a proliferation of mandatorily (and voluntarily)-fortified food products in the modern food supply. The nutrient intakes of more and more people are being influenced by the availability of these food products. So, where is food fortification headed?

Attempting to predict the future of food fortification is a fraught exercise because the social, economic, environmental, technological, and political determinants of public health will inevitably change and result in non-linear paths into the future. Nevertheless, insights from the case studies suggest that the antecedents (the dominant actors, activities, and agendas) behind the progressive growth in food fortification over the past century will continue to have an influential presence in public health policy deliberations into the future. Indeed, recent developments suggest that the 'stars are lining up' to facilitate a rapid expansion of food fortification interventions.

This chapter presents a brief overview of projections for food fortification interventions into the near future. This overview is followed by a discussion of three of the more powerful drivers behind this anticipated increased food fortification presence in the food supply into the future: new agendas, new investments, and new technologies. Drawing on findings from the research presented in this book, the chapter then suggests priority activities for managing food fortification as a technology for protecting and promoting public health.

Fortify, fortify, fortify

There are clear signs that the number of mandatory food fortification interventions and their coverage across populations is set to rapidly expand into the future. These signs include the: consolidation of current interventions; goals of pro-food fortification actors; and increasing number of staple foods that are being fortified, the number of added nutrients they contain, and their reach.

Consolidation of current interventions

Universal salt iodization (USI) has now achieved coverage of 70% of the world's population. Renewed efforts are underway to extend the proportion of the population covered by USI (3). Mandatory flour fortification with folic acid (MFFFA) has now been legislated in 66 countries (4). This number is set to almost certainly increase with the ongoing advocacy of the Flour Fortification Initiative (FFI) and the roll out of the Centers for Disease Control and Prevention's Global initiative to eliminate folic acid-preventable neural tube defects (5). Evidence associating vitamin D status with a range of potential health benefits is accumulating. A number of academics and medical practitioners are drawing on the evidence for these various health associations to advocate for mandatory milk fortification with vitamin D (MMFVD) as an intervention to help prevent specific diseases beyond bone health. For example, certain academics are advocating for the implementation of MMFVD in Scotland as an intervention to help reduce the prevalence of multiple sclerosis in that country (6).

Goals of pro-food fortification actors

FFI's 'aspirational goal' is for, '80% of the world's wheat flour from industrial mills to be fortified by 2015' (1). The Initiative reported in May 2012 a doubling in the number of countries with legislation mandating wheat flour fortification with at least iron or folic acid in eight years (7). GAIN's goal is to reach 1.5 billion people with fortified foods that have sustainable nutritional impact and it is continuing to expand its programmes and countries with which it is engaged to work towards this goal (2). These observations highlight the momentum that is underway for achieving the goals of these two prominent pro-food fortification actors.

Increasing number of staple foods that are being fortified, the number of added nutrients they contain, and their reach

Until recently the major food vehicles for wide-scale fortification programmes have been salt with iodine, oil with vitamin A, and wheat flour with iron and folic acid, and to a lesser extent foods such as milk and margarine with vitamin D. Now an increasing number of staple foods are being fortified. Wheat flour fortification interventions are being adapted for maize flour fortification and an increasing number of countries including the Philippines, Costa Rica, Papua, and Nicaragua are adopting rice fortification to tackle micronutrient malnutrition (8).

The number of nutrients being added to staple foods also has increased in recent years. For example, countries are being encouraged to extend wheat flour fortification beyond iron and folic acid to also include: vitamin A, zinc, vitamin D, vitamin B12, and other B vitamins such as thiamine, riboflavin, and niacin (9).

The ongoing growth in the industrial food system characterized by large-scale and centralized production and processing components and extensive distribution networks is providing a highly efficient mechanism for preparing and delivering fortified food products to maximize population reach.

Drivers of increased food fortification policy and practice into the future

New agendas

The Scaling Up Nutrition (SUN) agenda sets out a bold vision to address undernutrition, hunger, food and nutrition insecurity, and their consequences, particularly in low- and middle-income countries (LMICs) (10). As discussed in Chapter 8, SUN has high level support from governments around the world, United Nation (UN) agencies and leading public, private, and civil society organizations. In addition to encouraging governments to adopt national plans to scale up nutrition in their various sectoral policies, the SUN framework calls for the establishment of partnerships linking business, civil society, and government to foster scaling up nutrition through nutrition interventions at the country level. Such partnerships will provide increased capacity to expand global food fortification activities.

In relation to its investment in food fortification, the SUN agenda is faced with the challenge of balancing the expectations of actor's aligned with two contrasting approaches: an approach which promotes micronutrient interventions (supplementation and food fortification), and a human rights approach. The integral position of public–private partnerships (PPPs), and GAIN in particular, in the SUN initiative, will exert influence for food fortification interventions to receive particular attention in SUN activities. By contrast, in his report (11) submitted to the Human Rights Council in accordance with council resolution 13/4, the Special Rapporteur on the right to food stresses that the adoption of a human rights framework to promote adequate food should receive priority attention. This framework emphasizes investment in rebuilding and strengthening local food systems through diversified farming systems based on local knowledge and conditions, so that long term health and economic benefits can be achieved. Within this framework, food fortification is viewed as offering a short term solution to micronutrient malnutrition problems while local agrifood systems are being transformed to support local food production and economies.

New investments

The World Health Organization (WHO) is introducing new investments in technical and policy agendas to support food fortification interventions. Among its investments it is establishing a process for developing and updating evidence-informed guidelines for micronutrient interventions, preparing and commissioning systematic reviews of the evidence related to a particular intervention undergoing evaluation, upgrading and expanding its Vitamin and Mineral Nutrition Information System, and initiating research studies. WHO's investment in its electronic Library of Evidence for Nutrition Actions (eLENA) provides an expanding evidence catalogue for food fortification activities. The momentum underway is indicated by the outputs in the 2010–2011 biennium, a two-year period during which 16 evidence-informed guidelines for micronutrient interventions (mostly supplementation-related) were published, and new tools and resources were developed to support member states and their partners in implementing micronutrient interventions (12).

The investment in an expanded evidence base is being accompanied by new investments in advocacy activities. WHO is actively involved in advocating for food fortification through its activities to influence public policy and resource allocation decisions in a range of systems and institutions (12). In addition, a coalition of UN and private agencies has come together to advocate for increased investment in food fortification in a variety of settings (13).

New technologies

Nutrition science knowledge and technological developments are likely to continue to bolster the capabilities of scientists and food manufacturers to pursue food fortification on a large scale and with a variety of food vehicles.

Biofortification is a promising technology in this regard though more work is needed before its efficacy, effectiveness, and safety for humans and the environment is established. Biofortification of staple foods such as cereals, legumes, and tubers involves traditional crop breeding practices or transgenic techniques to improve the nutrient content and/or absorption of plants (14). A benefit of biofortification over conventional food fortification interventions is that the additional nutrient exposure is integrated into the food matrix suggesting physiological advantages (15). As with more conventional food fortification interventions a challenge will be the ability to manage such technologies so that they are a complement to public health programmes and not an imposition that might disrupt local food systems and economies.

Suggested priority activities for managing food fortification into the future

Into the future the momentum driving food fortification interventions shows little sign of abating. It is not possible to accurately predict the impact of burgeoning individual, and collective, food fortification interventions. However, planning can be put in place to manage potential benefits, risk and ethical considerations. In this regard and drawing on the insights obtained from the research presented throughout this book, the following priority activities are suggested for managing food fortification into the future as a technology to help protect and promote public health.

Policy priorities

A conceptual framework for placing expectations for food fortification interventions into perspective

The conventional orthodoxy for food fortification policy and practice is that evidential and ethical evaluative frameworks are used to inform food fortification policy-making (Chapter 2). These frameworks are important because they provide reasoning systems for decision-making. However, the case study findings have demonstrated that the decision-making process for food fortification interventions is not always rational. For a given public health nutrition policy problem there may be a number of potential policy solutions, including food fortification. When selecting from among policy options often there are competing views about what counts as evidence for assessing policy options and how ethical considerations might be justified.

A conceptual framework can strategically capture ways of thinking coherently and proactively about public health nutrition policy problems and the potential policy solutions available for their prevention and control. Central to a framework is the explicit identification of the underlying cause(s) of policy problems and how they relate to various policy options. Conceptualising a policy problem—policy solution relationship prompts policy-makers to think about evidence-informed policy in terms that extend beyond just considering the quantity and quality of evidence for a potential solution. Policy-makers are encouraged to also consider the 'relevance' of the evidence that is being used to inform policy. In this way a conceptual framework can place expectations about food fortification interventions and alternative policy options into perspective to help plan policy responses to the evidence of a policy problem. Politics and competing views are unlikely to be able to be removed from food fortification policy-making processes, but with a conceptual framework in place the thinking behind decisions is made more relevant and accountable.

Reform evidential and ethical evaluative frameworks

There has been much investment in developing the design and procedures for evidential evaluative frameworks. Yet the frameworks are not infallible. The case study investigations revealed that the frameworks have limitations in their nature and scope when applied to public health nutrition policy interventions, including food fortification. There is a need to reform how evidence of benefit is appraised, evidence of risk is analysed and ethics is considered in policy-making processes for such interventions.

Reforming the evidential approaches that currently are used to evaluate the effectiveness of a potential policy solution for a public health problem is indicated. Conventional approaches such as the 'Grading of recommendations assessment, development, and evaluation' methodology (Chapter 2) evolved from an evidence-based medicine background. Whereas these approaches are well suited to evaluating micronutrient interventions they struggle to accurately evaluate interventions that tackle the social, environmental and political determinants of public health problems. Approaches need to have the capability to extend beyond evaluating not just the quantity and quality of evidence for an intervention, but also the 'relevance' of the evidence for an intervention addressing a policy problem.

Reforming risk analysis frameworks also is indicated. The design of conventional risk analysis frameworks applied to public health nutrition interventions is based on an extension of a design founded in toxicology. The design has been adapted to accommodate certain nutrition characteristics and is well suited to analysing for relatively immediate health risks resulting from excessive nutrient intakes. However, its narrow scope restricts its ability to specify and measure the full range of potential public health implications associated with food fortification interventions. Risk analysis frameworks could consider the potential broader impacts of food fortification interventions on dietary imbalances as well as on environmental, economic and social outcomes, e.g. the potential to disrupt local food systems.

Reforming ethical evaluative frameworks is indicated in the sense that this investigation found few instances where ethics appeared to have been explicitly applied to food fortification policy-making processes. The application of an ethical justification process could be introduced into food fortification policy-making.

Research priorities

Increasing the evidence base for existing case studies

All investigated case studies were associated with scientific uncertainties. For example, the epidemiological evidence that informed MFFFA was convincing, yet the actual mechanism by which folic acid helps reduce the risk of neural tube defects is uncertain as is the optimum folic acid dose to exert this protective effect. Ongoing research is required to gain more evidence to elucidate these scientific uncertainties to help refine the planning and implementation of the case study interventions.

Increasing research investment into food fortification policy alternatives

Currently, a relatively large research investment is being directed towards conducting systematic reviews, cost-effective analyses and preparing policy guidelines for food fortification interventions. This is a positive development for informing policy processes for such interventions. However, an equivalent research investment to build the evidence base for alternative policy options, such as those consistent with a human rights approach, is required. Otherwise, policymakers will have a skewed evidence base to inform their decisions when selecting from among the policy options available to tackle public health problems.

Planning and implementation priorities

Food fortification democracy

Despite having their dietary intakes directly influenced by food fortification interventions, members of the public rarely are active participants in the decision-making processes that result in the proliferation of fortified foods in the marketplace. Instead they tend to be passive consumers of such products. The likelihood is that many people may be unaware of food fortification interventions affecting their nutrient intake as the presence of micrograms or even milligrams of added nutrients in fortified foods is not something that can be readily seen. Yet, with global health governance arrangements there is an increasing concentration of power over food fortification interventions and this power is resting with those with substantial resources to shape relevant policy-making processes.

Lessons can be drawn from Lang's argument that there is a need to invigorate a food democracy movement in which the public has greater involvement in food policy decision-making (16). Strengthening the democratic nature of governance arrangements that shape food fortification requires activities, consistent with health democracy activities in general. Specifically, it will require greater transparency in decision-making processes and support to promote the literacy and capacity of the public to participate in such processes (17). Ultimately the test of the success of such activities will be that food fortification is truly a demand-led and not supply-led, public health policy intervention.

Reforming global health governance arrangements

Complementing moves to democratize food fortification is the need to reform global health governance arrangements. In particular, PPPs are gaining more influence over policy-making processes and have changed the power relations between the public and private sectors in food fortification activities. Curiously, a relatively large amount of time is directed towards scrutinizing the formal mechanisms of the public sector in formulating food fortification interventions. Yet, relatively less time is spent scrutinizing the less transparent activities of business interest non-government organizations (BINGOs) and public interest non-government organizations (PINGOs) involved in food fortification activities. These organizations engage not only in various global health agendas with UN agencies but also enter into separate arrangements with individual countries and regions. The democratic principles followed by these organizations and their accountability are not always clear (18).

Concerns that have been levelled at the involvement of PPPs in health policy deliberations include: power imbalances among partners, whether inherent conflicts of interest are effectively managed, and the frequent failure to establish strong safeguards to protect public health goals from being co-opted by commercial interests (19). Important reforms that have been suggested to increase trust in PPPs include:

1 Separating policy formulation roles from policy implementation roles

Public health practitioners (20, 21) have argued that whereas there are benefits to be gained from involving BINGOs in policy implementation, it is not appropriate to involve them in policy formulation, especially in relation to the potential for a conflict of interest to arise. But it is not just BINGOs whose involvement in food fortification activities should be limited to policy implementation. A number of PINGOs engage with the private sector, e.g. the Micronutrient Initiative receives funding from Dow Chemical Company Foundation and Salt Institute, among others, and as such there can be a degree of overlap between how PINGOs and BINGOs might be managed in relation to issues such as potential conflicts of interest.

2 Evaluating the impacts of public–private partnerships

PPPs involved in food fortification activities are rarely independently evaluated. An important activity into the future will be to have independently evaluated the food fortification activities of organisations such as GAIN and FFI. Evaluations need to be inclusive of process measures such as transparency and participation (ability of alternative voices to be heard) as well as their impacts on nutrient intakes and health, economic, social, and environmental outcomes.

3 Strengthening accountability arrangements

Concerns have been expressed that current global health governance arrangements do not hold actors sufficiently accountable for their activities and that there is a need to develop standards for measuring success, monitoring progress and enforcement (22). A research team with whom the author is involved, examined the accountability of PPPs with food, beverage, and restaurant companies to address global hunger, undernutrition, and obesity. This research developed a benefit–risk decision-making pathway tool for prospective partners to assess partnership compatibility before engaging with industry and is a suggested priority activity for the public sector to incorporate into planning the involvement of PPPs with food fortification (23). The research also recommended that partners adopt systematic and transparent accountability processes to balance public health interests with private commercial interests, manage conflicts of interest, ensure that co-branded activities support food products that are consistent with dietary guidelines, comply with ethical codes of conduct, and monitor and evaluate partnership outcomes.

Monitoring and evaluation priorities

Undertaking food fortification monitoring and evaluation

The amount of work that is undertaken in researching, planning and implementing a food fortification intervention is rarely matched by its subsequent monitoring and evaluation (24). Without monitoring and evaluation activities being undertaken, it is not possible to know if an intervention is achieving its objectives. If it is not known if an intervention is achieving its objectives it is difficult to inform the ongoing development of the intervention and to learn from the experience to inform other food fortification interventions. Critically, practitioners need to be able to learn from food fortification failures as well as successes (25).

Into the future increased investment in monitoring and evaluation activities is needed so that data are collected on health outcomes, nutrition status, food consumption and composition data, on a comprehensive and timely basis to adequately inform food fortification policy processes. Food fortification monitoring and evaluation activities need to have the capacity to differentiate the relative contributions of mandatory food fortification, voluntary food fortification, dietary behaviour change, and supplementation to nutrition status and health outcomes. In addition it may be that the monitoring and evaluation needs to account for those situations where multiple food fortification interventions might be being implemented simultaneously. For instance, it is not inconceivable that different organizations operating in the same country could implement separate, non-coordinated micronutrient interventions where a nutrient such as iron might be added to more than one staple food as well as being promoted in supplemental form. An increased investment in monitoring and evaluation activities might be secured by making the approval of food fortification interventions conditional on demonstrated commitment to such activities.

Food fortification information systems

Underpinning food fortification policy-making is the need for a comprehensive and strategic food fortification information system. The case studies have revealed that it is not uncommon for a country to make a food fortification decision without sufficient evidence of the population's baseline nutrient intake, nutrition status, or policy problem prevalence. This situation raises ethical concerns about the decision-making process and it will make it difficult to evaluate interventions into the future. A food fortification information system should not only coordinate monitoring and evaluation activities, but also incorporate necessary mechanisms to enable collected information to be shared with the public, policy makers, and others involved in food fortification interventions in a timely and ongoing basis. An efficient information system should build in milestones and requirements for reviewing the evidence that emerges from the monitoring and evaluation to then increase accountability and feedback findings into the ongoing review of the intervention.

References

1. Flour Fortification Initiative. [cited 8 October 2012]. Available from: http://www. ffinetwork.org/about/index.html.

2. Global Alliance for Improved Nutrition. *About GAIN*. 2011 [cited 23 March 2012]. Available from: http://www.gainhealth.org/about-gain.

3. WHA. *WHA 63/27:A63/27, Progress reports—Sustaining the elimination of iodine deficiency disorders (WHA60.21), Geneva, 15 April* 2010. Geneva: World Health Organization; 2010 [cited 26 April 2012]. Available from: http://www.who.int/ nutrition/topics/A63.27_idd_en.pdf.

4. Lawrence M, Kripalani K. Profiling national mandatory folic acid fortification policy around the world. In: Preedy V (ed). *Handbook of food fortification and health: from concepts to public health applications*. New York: Springer; in press.

5. CDC. *Global initiative to eliminate folic acid-preventable neural tube defects*. [cited 29 May 2012]. Available from: http://www.cdc.gov/ncbddd/folicacid/global.html.

6. Boseley S. Add vitamin D to Scotland's food – experts. *The Guardian* 2011; 23 December. [cited 8 October 2012]. Available from: http://www.guardian.co.uk/ uk/2011/dec/23/vitamin-d-scotland-food-multiple-sclerosis.

7. Flour Fortification Initiative. *Number of countries with fortification legislation doubles in eight years*. [cited 4 June 2012]. Available from: http://www.sph.emory.edu/ wheatflour/68_Countries.pdf.

8. Global Alliance for Improved Nutrition. *RiFoRG. Rice fortification frequently asked questions*. [cited 4 June 2012]. Available from: http://www.gainhealth.org/riforg/sites/ default/files/RiFoRG_FAQs_Jan%202011.pdf.

9. Flour Fortification Initiative. [cited 4 June 2012]. Available from: http://www.sph. emory.edu/wheatflour/effects.php.

10. United Nations System Standing Committee on Nutrition. *Scaling Up Nutrition: A Framework for Action. Based on a series of consultations hosted by the Center for Global Development, the International Conference on Nutrition, USAID, UNICEF and the World Bank*; 2010.

11. United Nations General Assembly Human Rights Council. *Report submitted by the Special Rapporteur on the right to food, Oliver De Schutter. Nineteenth session. A/HRC/19/59. Agenda item 3*. 26 December 2011. Geneva: United Nations; 2011 [cited 8 October 2012]. Available from: http://www2.ohchr.org/english/bodies/ hrcouncil/docs/19session/A.HRC.19.59_English.pdf.

12. World Health Organization. *WHO, Draft Report, Micronutrients 2010–2011, WHO/NMH/NHD/EPG/12.1*. Geneva: Department of Nutrition for Health and Development; 2011.

13. Micronutrient Initiative. *Micronutrient Initiative, Investing in the future: A united call to action on vitamin and mineral deficiencies, Global report* 2009 [cited 8 October 2012]. Available from: http://www.unitedcalltoaction.org.

14. Bouis HE, Hotz C, McClafferty B, Meenakshi JV, Pfeiffer WH. Biofortification: a new tool to reduce micronutrient malnutrition. *Food and Nutrition Bulletin* 2011; 32(1 Suppl):S31–40.

15. Wahlqvist M. National food fortification: a dialogue with reference to Asia: policy in evolution. *Asia Pacific Journal of Clinical Nutrition* 2008; 17(Suppl 1):24–9.

16. Lang T. Food industrialisation and food power: Implications for food governance. *Development Policy Review* 2003; 21(5):555–68.

17. Lofgren H, de Leeuw E, Leahy M (eds). *Democratizing Health: Consumer groups in the policy process*, Edward Elgar, Cheltenham; 2011.

18. Kraak V, Swinburn B, Lawrence M, Harrison P. The accountability of public-private partnerships with food, beverage and restaurant companies to address global hunger and the double burden of malnutrition. *SCN News. Nutrition and Business: How to Engage?* 2011; 39:11– 24 [cited 3 June 2012]. Available from: http://www. unscn.org/files/Publications/SCN_News/SCNNEWS39_10.01_high_def.pdf.

19. Buse K, Harmer A. Seven habits of highly effective global public-private health partnerships: practice and potential. *Social Science and Medicine* 2007; 64(2):259–71.

20. Brady M, Rundall P. *Governments should govern, and corporations should follow the rules*. 2011 [cited 8 October 2012]. Available from: http://www.unscn.org/files/Publications/SCN_News/SCNNEWS39_10.01_high_def.pdf.

21. Gomes F, Lobstein T. Food and beverage transnational corporations and nutrition policy, In: *SCN News. Nutrition and Business: How to Engage?* 2011; 39:51–6.

22. Gostin L, Friedman E, Ooms G, Gebauer T, Gupta N, Sridhar D, *et al.* The Joint Action and Learning Initiative: towards a global agreement on national and global responsibilities for health. *PLoS Medicine* 2011; 8(5):e1001031.

23. Kraak V, Harrigan P, Lawrence M, Harrison P, Jackson M, Swinburn B. Balancing the benefits and risks of public-private partnerships to address the global double burden of malnutrition. *Public Health Nutrition* 2011; 15(3):503–17.

24. Allen L, de Benoist B, Dary O, Hurrell R. *Guidelines on food fortification with micronutrients*. Geneva: World Health Organization; 2006 [cited 8 October 2012]. Available from: http://www.who.int/nutrition/publications/guide_food_fortification_micronutrients.pdf.

25. Yngve A, Haapala I, Allison Hodge, Geraldine McNeill, Marilyn Tseng. "Interpreting success and failure in food fortification." *Public Health Nutrition* 2012; 15(10):1789–90.

Chapter 10

Conclusion

Food fortification can be a powerful technology for protecting and promoting public health. It has a history of successfully being used to tackle public health nutrition problems caused by an inherent nutrient deficiency in the food supply. In recent times, mandatory food fortification is increasingly being adopted in various countries to tackle public health nutrition problems caused by social-economic (micronutrient malnutrition) and primarily genetic (neural tube defects (NTDs)) circumstances, as well as those caused by certain living conditions and cultural, religious, and social customs (vitamin D deficiency). As a policy solution for these problems, the adoption of food fortification can be controversial.

Advances in nutrition knowledge and food science capabilities are contributing to mandatory food fortification becoming more widespread and being implemented using an increasing number of food vehicles and variety of nutrient combinations. In lieu of the increasing use and presence of food fortification interventions, public health policy-makers and practitioners need to be critically aware of how best to manage this technology to protect and promote public health. The research presented in this book has drawn attention to food fortification policy and practice being intertwined with debates about evidence, ethics, and politics. In this conclusion to the book, the case study findings are generalized to food fortification in total and then used to identify lessons for food fortification evidence and food fortification politics.

Generalizing the case study findings to food fortification in total

The frame of reference for the research presented in this book was food fortification as a technology for public health nutrition policy. It is to food fortification in total that the findings from each of the three case studies are generalized. Each case study was selected as being representative of a particular policy problem aligned with one of three plausible food fortification rationales. The case study findings showed that universal salt iodization (USI) 'performed' well as an intervention to help prevent and control iodine deficiency disorders. Therefore, it would be predicted that mandatory food fortification is a highly

recommended intervention when the food supply is unable to provide sufficient nutrients because of an inherent nutrient deficiency in the food supply.
Mandatory flour fortification with folic acid (MFFFA) and mandatory milk
fortification with vitamin D (MMFVD) performed less well in preventing neural tube defects and vitamin D deficiency, respectively. Therefore, mandatory
food fortification is generally not highly recommended when the rationale for
adding nutrients to the food supply is that certain individuals have nutrient
requirements higher than reference standards or when there is a reduction in
exposure to the primary source of a nutrient. However, these findings were
qualified for certain situations. In the situation of helping prevent and control
anaemia resulting from a medical condition affecting a significant number of
individuals, mandatory food fortification with iron is recommended. Also
MMFVD is recommended when implemented strategically as a component of
a multifaceted program.

Food fortification evidence and ethics

It might be asked that if the primary objective in food regulation is the protection of public health and safety, 'Why might there be public health and ethical
concerns with food fortification interventions if this objective is observed?'.
The answer is that the objective is not clearly defined as such and takes on
meaning through the application of evaluative frameworks that are designed to
assess the evidence for public health benefits and risks of food fortification.
What counts as evidence and how ethics is viewed is socially constructed.
Typically, the frameworks are being constructed from a reductionist view of
food and health relationships. This orthodoxy works well when assessing relationships between a single nutrient and a specific biological outcome, as is the
case with USI. However, the relationships between public health nutrition
problems and their potential solutions often are more complex, as is the case
with most micronutrient malnutrition problems. The evaluative frameworks
are not well designed to specify and measure complex relationships. For this reason their assessment of public health benefits and risks tends to privilege micronutrient interventions (supplementation, fortification) over alternative public
health nutrition policy interventions. This research has highlighted that generally
the management of food fortification is taking place in the absence of a conceptual analysis of the nature and causes of public health nutrition problems.

Into the future, it will be important that evaluative frameworks are reformed
so that they are responsive to the nature of a public health nutrition problem
being investigated. This means that the frameworks need to appraise all relevant evidence for public health interventions and not just that which conforms
with a rigid schema. The insight that emerged from this research was the need

for evaluative frameworks to conceptualize a policy problem by considering its causation. Taking causation into account will result in the evaluative frameworks' assessment of policy responses being more relevant to the problem at hand. For example, the effectiveness of policy options to tackle micronutrient malnutrition will vary depending on whether the cause of this problem is poverty or an inherent nutrient deficiency in the food supply. Evaluative frameworks need flexibility to adapt to either circumstance.

Mandatory food fortification interventions increase the nutrient intake of everyone in the population who consumes the fortified food. This characteristic raises significant ethical considerations. Yet, there were few instances where ethical justification was apparent in policy-making processes. It is situations like this that highlight the need for greater inclusion of an ethical justification procedure in evaluative frameworks during the assessment of mandatory food fortification interventions.

Food fortification politics

Food fortification has a powerful impact on food composition, food systems, food economies and public health. Inevitably, many actors have a stake in the development of food fortification activities. The case study findings highlighted the inherently political nature of food fortification. Science and technology may provide the capability to fortify foods, but their use is frequently contested among actors with opposing values, beliefs, and interests towards food and health relationships. Ultimately, it is political processes and judgements that determine if, when, how, and why this capability might be translated into food fortification policy and practice.

The policy process varied across the case studies, but for all case studies it was informed to a certain extent by evidence (and sometimes ethics). Nevertheless, the lesson that emerges for the food fortification policy process in general is that evidence and ethics do not speak for themselves in the policy-making process. The way evidence and ethics are constructed, interpreted, and applied is political—it is influenced by the interplay of actors, their activities, and dominant political agendas. Fundamentally, food fortification policies and practices reflect the policy environment within which they are made. In the current global policy-making environment, powerful coalitions of actors are promoting food fortification with strategic advocacy and framing activities and supported by global health governance arrangements that in particular are privileging public–private partnerships and their food fortification agendas.

It is not the intention of this research to reject evidence- and ethics-informed food fortification policy because it is as an unattainable ideal. It remains an ideal to which to aspire. Achieving this ideal will require improvements in the transparency of policy-making and the opportunity for those affected by food fortification activities to have a greater say in the policy processes.

Into the future, food fortification policy and practice will continue to be a dynamic area. As the evidence base evolves, the case for USI, MFFFA, and MMFVD may change. In the meantime there is momentum for increasing their population coverage globally, e.g. with the Scaling Up Nutrition initiative there is likely to be a greater investment in food fortification to tackle micronutrient malnutrition. In addition, calls for new food fortification applications are likely to arise as evidence for public health nutrition problems emerges. As food progressively becomes more and more a carrier of novel amounts and mixtures of added nutrients its composition will depart further from that with which humans have evolved. Ongoing monitoring and evaluation of the impact of individual and collective food fortification activities on the nutrient composition of foods, population nutrient intakes, health outcomes, and food system operations, will be critical to inform policy and practice to protect and promote public health.

Index